PERIOD QUEEN

Published in 2020 by Murdoch Books, an imprint of Allen & Unwin

Murdoch Books Australia
83 Alexander Street, Crows Nest NSW 2065
Phone: +61 (0)2 8425 0100
murdochbooks.com.au
info@murdochbooks.com.au

Murdoch Books UK
Ormond House, 26–27 Boswell Street, London WC1N 3JZ
Phone: +44 (0) 20 8785 5995
murdochbooks.co.uk
info@murdochbooks.co.uk

Publisher: Jane Morrow
Editorial Manager: Julie Mazur Tribe
Design Manager: Megan Pigott
Editor: Katie Bosher
Designer and illustrator: Ngaio Parr
Production Manager: Megan Cosgrove
Cover design by Alissa Dinallo
Cover illustrations by Ngaio Parr

ISBN 978 1 76052 508 8 Australia
ISBN 978 1 91163 246 7 UK

 A catalogue record for this book is available from the National Library of Australia

A catalogue record for this book is available from the British Library

Printed and bound in Australia by Griffin Press

10 9 8 7 6 5 4 3

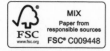 The paper in this book is FSC® certified. FSC® promotes environmentally responsible, socially beneficial and economically viable management of the world's forests.

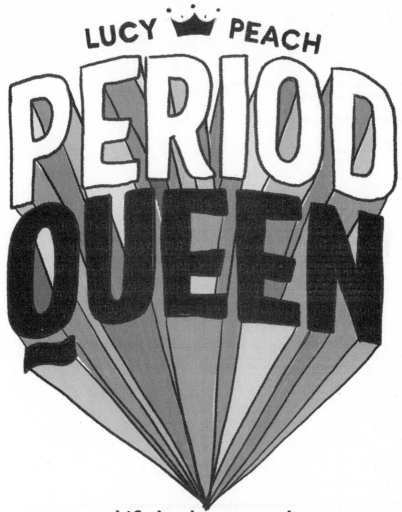

LUCY 👑 PEACH

PERIOD QUEEN

Life hack your cycle
and own your power
all month long

murdoch books
Sydney | London

CONTENTS

WELCOME

This book takes the 'worst thing' about being a woman and restores it to the best thing. It will teach you to harness the four powers of your menstrual cycle. If I really had to, I could sum up the whole idea in about fifteen words and six seconds with this:

Hey you! Your period is bloody awesome, now go live your best life! The end.

We live in an age where there are whole industries dedicated to helping us find balance and direction. Yet the greatest life hack of them all is right under our noses (or rather belly buttons) and it isn't knowing how to perfectly execute a blackhead removal or disguise the taste of kale in a smoothie, *it's your menstrual cycle.* We've channelled solar power, wind power and even tidal power, now it's time for us to channel menstrual power. You already have all the balance and direction you need; you just need to tune in and learn how to use it.

In an ideal world, I wouldn't even need to write this book because everything in it would already be common knowledge — just like the changing seasons, night and day or the Earth being round. Menstrual wisdom would be passed down with pride and spoken of openly as the absolutely normal thing it is. We would learn to respect the hormonal changes that we experience throughout the month, and as a result the notion that having female hormones reduces us to being random emotional roller-coasters would grind to a halt and rust away into oblivion.

We would feel less overwhelmed, frustrated and/or inadequate because the rest of the world wouldn't be so fixated on everyone being the same *Every. Single. Day.* We would experience slow days and fast days, days more about looking after others and days more about looking after ourselves, and we'd rest assured that by going with the flow (literally) it would all come out in the wash.

It would be normal to track your cycle and to notice — and, more importantly, to use — the benefits that it brings. Yes, you read that right: there are useful benefits.

We'd be more inclined to ~~like~~ *love* ourselves, all month long. We'd have an unwavering trust in our intuition. Can you imagine?

Boys would learn about cycles and grow up to be men who appreciate the benefits of being attuned to them. Men would also be afforded the benefits of going with their own flow, and together we would find a balance between masculine and feminine, breathe a collective sigh of relief and voilà: we'd embrace the tides, love our bodies and their life-giving hormones, and ride unicorns into the horizon towards world peace and harmony.

This book is a public service announcement to address a long-held astronomical misunderstanding about menstruation. It's called a 'cycle' for a reason, and the truth is it's *so* much more than the presence or absence of your period and how to 'manage' it. You don't need to push through the hormonal ups and downs, holding on for dear life, because there *is* a better way, and it's pretty bloody amazing. Please observe.

Every month, you have four hormonal phases.

They each arrive in turn, one after the other, bearing their own gifts and ways of making us feel. And once you know what they are, you can predict them, plan for them and *use* them over and over again. I guarantee that if you get to the bottom of how truly marvellous you are in every phase, you will be UNSTOPPABLE (except, of course, when you choose to stop). Before you know it, you will have developed your own cycle superpowers.

I have no doubt that a league of truly empowered women who are fiercely aware that everything about their bodies happens for a reason is precisely what this planet desperately needs. Like an alarm that's been left snoozing for thousands of years, the Earth's whispers are growing to an exasperated roar: 'HEY, GIRLS! LADIES? ANYONE? Are your arms and legs painted on? Your exceptional powers are *needed*.'

Wake up, World!

I'm not saying it will always be easy or that you'll cycle through life farting rainbows and sprinkling stardust with the demeanour of the Dalai Lama. Life will still disappoint you sometimes; that's an undeniable fact. But when it does, you won't have to face it alone and you'll be able to catch yourself before you roll around in it (the disappointment) like a dog with something smelly. You will become an expert in recognising what you need at different times of the month. Hard things won't seem quite as hard anymore because you'll be able to hold them up to the light and see them through the all-knowing lens of your cycle. This connection to your body is like a compass, always there for you and waiting, *wanting*, to guide you back to balance.

With every cycle, you have a chance to cultivate the most important relationship of your life: the one with your precious self. This relationship lasts for *your entire life*, and certainly long after your bleeding stops. That is the power of the period, how you cycle like a queen and the point of this book.

To that end, welcome to this manual for the art of harnessing the four menstrual cycle superpowers. Stay with me and all will become clear as we uncover how they can affect us hormonally, physically and emotionally. I'll be speaking as someone who's had approximately 300 cycles of my own, as well as years of experience as a sexual health educator, a human biology teacher and a period preacher.

This moment in time has been thousands of years in the making, and I'm so glad that, at long last, you are I are on this same page together because once you understand the powers you've been born with, you can *use* them: for good, for bad or whatever you bleeding well like because they're yours. Knowing and speaking of this power is your birthright, and I'm excited for you and all you will discover as you start to apply it to your excellent self.

For everyone with a menstrual cycle, this book is for you. If you plan on having one in the future, this book is for you. This book is also for you if you don't have a cycle but you know someone who does and want to better support them and understand what makes them tick. What greater gift could you give — to yourself, to someone you know, or even a complete stranger? So read on, dear legend, whomever you are: this book *is* for you, this book is for everyone. It's time to give the menstrual cycle the long overdue rebrand it's been waiting for. Everyone needs to know the good news:

The future is bloody awesome.

HOW TO USE THIS BOOK

If you're chomping at the bit to read about your menstrual superpowers, feel free to jump ahead to page 62. Otherwise, carry on to find out how I came to be a period preacher and why we need this book so badly, and for a quick biology lesson on how our incredible bodies work.

HOW i CAME TO BE A PERIOD PREACHER

I am from Perth, Western Australia (WA), where the Whadjuk people of the Noongar nation have lived and cared for the land for over 60,000 years. I was born in 1980 — at a time of immense change for women. Thanks to the Whitlam government of the early 1970s, payments were introduced so single mothers (like mine) could afford to keep their children. There was action against discrimination, legislation to ensure pay equity, restrictions lifted on the sale of contraception and funding was allocated for women's refuges and health centres.

These are things we take for granted now, but when I was a baby and my mother was still a girl, they changed everything — especially for us. It was the beginning of a new world, and in it, we grew up together.

When she calls to wish me a happy birthday, I say, 'Thanks for having me, Mum.' And I really mean it. I imagine her at seventeen, determined, brave, surrounded by a sisterhood and pregnant with me.

At twelve, on my last day of primary school, she bought me new jeans from Myer. We were on our way to the airport. I'd never been on a plane or away from her, and now I was bound for London to spend the holidays with my dad. As she hugged me goodbye, I was excited — maybe a little nervous; I'd only met him once, two years before.

On account of being twelve, I was flying as an unaccompanied minor, so I got special attention from the flight attendants; my meals were served first and I was given little packets of paper and pencils. I busied myself on the long-haul flight by watching *The Bodyguard*, drinking Coke, filing my nails and writing in my journal. I had never in my life felt so sophisticated.

Just before we landed in Malaysia for the stopover, I went to the tiny bathroom and discovered that I had gotten my period. My period! I wanted to poke my head out of the cubicle door and announce, 'Hey! I'm a *WOMAN!*' At the very least I wanted to notify the attendant that I would no longer be requiring any special assistance because I was, after all, a bleeding lady, going *international*.

With my head high and my shoulders back (and complimentary pads stuffed into my pockets), I walked back to my seat thinking, *I am a woman. I'm an actual woman now. This must be how it feels. Just like this.* I continued watching Whitney Houston and Kevin Costner, content with my newly minted womanhood as I dinged the bell for more celebratory Coke. Maybe it felt so momentous because I was already on such an adventure — mid-air above the Indian Ocean en route to a dad I didn't actually know. It felt like a rite of passage that I was ready for.

This beautiful traditional Native American proverb befit the moment: 'At her first bleeding a woman meets her power. During her bleeding years she practises it. At menopause she becomes it.'

So there, at 30,000 feet, I met my power. And I did feel it then: a delicious secret hidden in my belly (as well as an ache in my lower back later, while I wandered through every museum and gallery in London with my dad). But soon, like all the other girls I came to know, the extent of my connection with my period was reduced to the barest facts: I knew when I was having it (obviously), I knew when I wasn't and I worried when it was late. I never imagined for a moment that my menstrual cycle could be remotely advantageous, other than as an excuse to avoid sport. I just didn't think about it that much.

What was this 'power' the Native Americans spoke about? And what did it have to do with my period?

I wouldn't find out for another 180 periods.

Fifteen years after my first period, while working as a sexual health educator at Family Planning WA (now known as Sexual Health Quarters, or SHQ), I learned the names and symptoms of every single sexually transmitted infection. I learned how to talk to little kids about puberty and to fourteen-year-olds about contraception and enthusiastic consent. I spoke with refugee women, boys in prison, girls with intellectual disabilities, youth workers, health workers and parents, and I relished the opportunity to create moments of empowerment, openness and positivity.

If I ever had questions about my body, I had plenty of people to ask. I learned (joy of joys) that I could request to insert my own speculum for a pap smear and have the test results sent to my home address.

I spent a lot of time in the largest sexual health library in the Southern Hemisphere, and I read furiously. Everything. I knew how lucky I was to be getting paid to absorb such a wealth of information that not only educated and empowered me, but also informed the way I parented, cared for myself and conducted myself in relationships and the world. And while I was reading and learning all of this new information at home, my little son would snuggle up to me and look at the pictures. His favourite bedtime story was a pregnancy manual, and when he asked me questions, I answered him honestly.

I had different bags in the back seat of my car for different school education sessions, filled with banana penis models, condoms and STIs as soft toys. If you ever saw a woman driving down the Kwinana Freeway with a toddler casually pointing a speculum out of the back window pretending to shoot people, that was me.

Every morning at work, I would learn things I didn't know I didn't know just by walking past the display stand in the library on the way to my desk. I'll never forget seeing the cover of *The Optimized Woman* by Miranda Gray. I picked it up and began to read it on the spot. That was the moment I discovered the bleeding obvious: I live in a linear world but *I'm not actually linear.* I'm cyclical. Duh. And so is half of the population. It was the biggest light-bulb moment of my life to date, and I stood there, rooted to the spot, making a mental note to tell everyone I knew.

No wonder I sometimes felt frustrated, overwhelmed, inadequate or like I was completely nailing life one minute and then having the rug pulled out from under me the next. I live in a world set up to cater to the biology of men, which is the same every day. This is a world that expects and rewards linear behaviour, and demands that women must push through their months despite the fact that our biology is completely different and always changing. Talk about a square peg in a round hole!

My mind was blown. Not just because this was revolutionary to *me*, but because I couldn't believe that no one had ever told me anything about this before! Could it be that no one I knew actually knew about it? This idea seemed impossible because what I'd learned felt too important and too useful. Too powerful.

I wanted to roar when I realised how long I'd spent doubting myself and how, as a young woman, I'd often dismissed my feelings as 'just my hormones'. How much I had diminished myself. Up until then, I'd congratulate myself when I felt that I was nailing life. *Look at me go. I'm nailing it! Now I just have to stay this way!* I viewed those 'easy weeks' as flukes and then felt frustrated and disappointed when, inevitably, I couldn't keep it up. I hadn't seen the pattern. I thought it was just me not nailing life enough.

Although I had long held my actual period in a fairly positive regard, I hadn't seen it as part of a cycle. Once I understood it, I began paying attention to myself. *Really* paying attention. I began paying attention to how and when I changed throughout the month, and instead of perceiving my fluidity as a weakness or an inadequacy, I came to see it as a strength. The more I noticed this, the more I noticed that at different times of the month, I just had different strengths.

I started seeing myself, and my whole life, through a new lens. Before giving myself a hard time (as was my previous default response), I would check where I was in my cycle and ask myself two simple questions:

What day am I on?

What do I most need right now?

It was such a relief not to feel as much pressure to be the same all month long. My manager at the sexual health clinic was excited about the benefits, too. She'd ask, 'So, which phase are you in now?' and then she'd factor in where we were both at before planning meetings or beginning new projects. If I felt tired during my period, I'd have a nap in the spare room during my lunch break or go home a little earlier and make up the time the following week, when I had extra energy in the tank. After noticing how I moved through the phases of my cycle, I began to plan for them and to really use them.

It made so much sense to me to live this way — it just made me feel more like *me*. I told anyone who'd listen, preaching period power with all the fervour of a new convert, and it seemed there was no end to the ways that I could apply it. I discovered that I could use certain phases as a creative tool for my already established songwriting, and, later, to navigate my way through a difficult break-up, to better teach, parent, be a friend and, most of all, to love myself.

MY GREATEST PERIOD EVER!

Fast forward to a windy afternoon about 100 cycles later while at Wedge Island, a tiny remote fishing-shack community in the middle of a national park on the Western Australian coast. I was making a music video with my creative director husband Richard, an assistant, a videographer and a florist.

'Hmm,' I mused, trying to make out my reflection in a filthy mirror, 'which scarf and which lipstick for this scene? F%ck it. Hot pink. I am in my ovulatory phase, after all.'

Alan Gilrod was our assistant on the shoot. He'd been a clown in Cirque du Soleil and was now stretched out on an old, rusty bed frame. He lifted his head and asked with an incredulous expression, 'What? What *are* you talking about? What is this phase?' I finished applying my lipstick and configuring my head-scarf while giving him a synopsis of what it meant to understand and live through your cycle.

All the while, he was agape. 'You need to make a show about this!' he spluttered. 'Do it! Do it and I'll help you!' Alan was already producing some shows for Perth Fringe Festival and offered to produce mine, too.

I took it as a dare. I saw the whole show instantly laid out in my mind: it would be just like a sex-ed session, only all about life hacking your period! It would be just like a gig but with more stories. And it would have . . . capes! 'OK!' I exclaimed. 'I will!' But then I caught myself. 'Actually, back up Alan. I'm in the phase where I say yes to everything. Can I give it a week and think about it?' When even my premenstrual self was committed, I knew it was the right thing for me to do.

While I wrote the show, Richard was the perfect sounding board. He'd make positive noises whenever I sat upright in bed with an idea, and he was the one who came up with the title: *My Greatest Period Ever*. I practised it over and over in front of my then eleven-year-old son. He told me which bits were funny and which bits needed more work, explaining or eliminating. Finally, a few days before opening night, I rehearsed the show in front of Richard, who said, 'Luce, it's fantastic. Really, it's great.'

'But what?' I asked, sensing his hesitation.

'Well, I'm just thinking that if you had all the time and money in the world, you could really do some fantastic visuals. You have some pretty complicated concepts in there, and maybe a few diagrams would help people to understand them better?'

I sighed loudly. 'Well, I have neither of those things [time or money], and the show starts in three days. What if you just drew me some quick diagrams?'

Asking a creative to 'just do a quick' anything is like waving a red rag in front of a bull, but Richard's not one to deny a challenge or a chance to make me happy. He agreed to give it a go, and we sat on the couch together and ran through the entire show, me talking and singing, Richard drawing in a scrapbook.

On opening night, he joined me for the show, sitting left of stage and scribbling furiously onto an iPad that was projected onto a screen. I talked quickly and he struggled to keep up, but even his crap drawings were so bad they were good. People loved that the show was not only about empowerment through the menstrual cycle, but that there was this man literally animating his wife's menstrual musings, sitting quietly in the corner while I sang and gave out capes and chocolate.

We sold out the entire run of shows, and the reception was incredible. Women and girls came in pairs and small gangs, and then they'd come back the following nights with their male partners and friends, saying to them, 'YOU have to know this, too!' The buzz was palpable, and every night after we finished, theatre management scolded us because our audience took so long to leave that the next act had trouble getting in. People gathered in the foyer and talked excitedly to each other and to complete strangers about their periods — even our lighting technician, who'd been visibly less than impressed with the content of the show at our first meeting, caught the buzz. After the final performance, he said, 'I really get it. I can't believe how much this makes sense!' He looked sheepish for a moment then added, 'It actually made me wish . . . that I had a period!' This was, and still is, a major career highlight for me. But it was just the beginning.

My Greatest Period Ever won the top prize, the Martin Sims award for the Best Western Australian production, and we were given $10,000 to take the show to the Brighton Fringe Festival in the UK. I was invited to speak at two TEDx appearances, and the following year we did the Melbourne Comedy Festival and the Sydney Fringe Festival for a string of sold-out shows.

We reimagined a version of the show for a younger audience and called it *How to Period Like a Unicorn*. The night before our last unicorn show, I'd been booked to play an acoustic set at Mia Freedman's book launch. I invited her along and she came. The next morning over breakfast, she gave me the most valuable advice: 'Woman! Write a book!'

WHY WE NEED THIS BOOK SO BADLY

One could spend years uncovering the stones and then turning them over for clues as to how exactly periods came to be so incredibly hushed and hidden. Our most tender and ancient magic, buried. This is an important exercise but I'm impatient to get to the good bits, and instinct tells me that I should cut to the chase: we need this book because we don't have nearly enough period pride yet. We need it because periods are still used as an insult and to cause shame. We need it because women are taught how to 'manage' periods with various blood-catching options (if we're lucky), then sent on our merry way without so much as a mud map for the entire hormonal and emotional landscape that accompanies a menstrual cycle. I feel FURIOUS that people aren't told the full story, that they grow up thinking the menstrual cycle is just like an on and off switch or some wild, unpredictable thing that is beyond comprehension (and that then, by extension, so are WE). We have a lot of ground to make up.

It's completely understandable if you've ever felt betrayed by your body — exasperated even. Indeed, most of us (including me) have idly thought at some point, *Just why? Why on earth does my vagina have to bleed? Is this some kind of design flaw? Who can I blame? God? Goddess? Come on.*

Irrespective of the evolutionary pathway that led us to period, our feelings towards it are further hampered because for an extremely long time we haven't exactly sold the concept very well. In fact, if it were a product, the slogan would be, 'Menstrual cycle: world's worst seller. Free* to a good home. You pick up.'

So how did we get here? Why are periods seen as nature's booby prize? To understand why this book is so necessary and why it's time we learn about periods differently, we need to take a look at how we've learned about them in the past and currently still do.

Except, actually not free at all and, depending on where and how you live and the privileges you have or don't, it can really cost you to have a period: physically, emotionally, socially and financially.

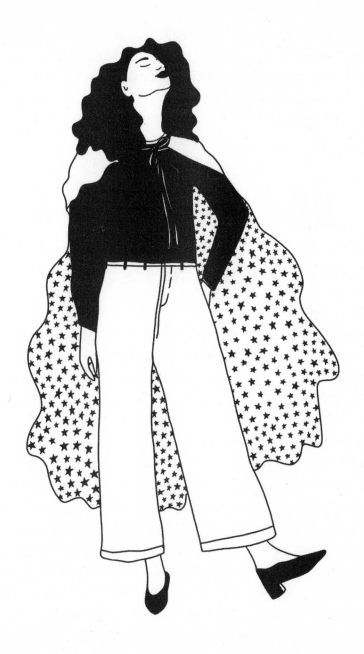

CHAPTER 1

HOW WE LEARN TO 'GIRL'

In Year 7 I had a crush on a boy with red hair and freckles. One day, he was pinching things out of my pencil case and I told him, indignantly, with my hands on my hips that he'd better stop it or else I'd blow my top. He smiled cheekily and said, 'I'd like to see that.' I was inwardly thrilled. I remember looking down at my yellow T-shirt and admiring myself in it, in agreement. It felt good.

Later, during a perfunctory health session, girls and boys were separated and told about menstrual management or erections and wet dreams, respectively. Already, it felt like we girls were getting the rough end of the stick. Periods meant babies, so naturally sex ed soon followed, which was mainly a course in disaster management, what with pregnancy, STIs and our reputations to worry about. No mention was made of pleasure, and there was an absence of positivity and diversity around what 'sex' could mean. There was an implication that boy bodies were built for pleasure while ours would yield discomfort, waste and the potential for life-altering risks. Somewhere along the way, I learned that pleasure was less about something I could feel and more about what I was able, or expected, to provide. Pleasure wasn't assumed.

My initial foray into my sexuality was overshadowed by attention I didn't want, or ask for, from men. In between worlds, wanting to be seen and to express myself but also simultaneously horrified. With a mixture of pride and mortification, my friends and I would reel off how many times we had been catcalled, leered at, offered a lift or had some vague 'compliment' yelled at us while walking to school that morning. We were in Year 8. I learned to walk with my eyes lowered and my arms crossed, and I associated this part of myself more with pressure than with pleasure. So observed was I in my growing body, that sometimes I wanted to disappear altogether.

I felt no agency over my sexuality, and I saw sex as something best gotten out of the way. Everyone said it was normal that it would hurt. But what if a girl knew of the pleasure she deserved because first she'd learned how to give it to herself? Would she be as inclined to explore her sexuality with someone she didn't feel safe with?

This ethos reflects the approach in the Netherlands, where children are taught about their bodies in an open and positive way from a very young age. Studies have shown that as a result, they are likely to begin having sex later than youth in other Western countries, and the most common reason given for having sex was 'they were in love'. Whether this is true for a week or a year or five minutes doesn't matter as much as the positivity of their experience. Young people in similar Australian studies talked more about the presence of alcohol and pressure from a partner. Today's young people also learn about sexuality in the context of porn, which can interfere with the more human and accidental ways to discover and explore. At the very least, girls need to learn about their own biology because the reality of the pleasure we are innately capable of, in partnership or alone, is a wonderous thing.

The clitoris. It is the only part of a human body (male or female) designed specifically for pleasure, and it's a far cry from the innocent little nub shown in anatomy diagrams. Incredibly, biologists didn't even know what the complete organ for female pleasure looked like until 2009, many years after the far more complex human genome had been mapped. I suggest you jump online immediately and search '3D model of the clitoris' to see for yourself a complete map of the organ dedicated to erotic sensation in the female body. You'll see that this little pea-sized nub is actually the tip of a miraculous wishbone-shaped iceberg. Fancy telling girls how to use period products but omitting this lovely bit of anatomy!

Every girl should know of her innate capacity for pleasure; even if she does (or you do), it can still be a very confusing time, but learning about your sexuality and exploring it safely is an important part of learning how to girl (along with climbing trees and frying eggs). Learn what you like, what you don't, and most importantly, learn how to voice it and speak openly. Ask questions, of your partners, your friends, of the women you trust, but for the best advice, always listen to your intuition.

THE SECRET SHAME CLUB

Eventually, we learn that periods are normal enough except for the small fact that they are practically unmentionable: not to be spoken of in public and under no circumstances around boys or men. Our blood might offend them or make them uncomfortable. It might remind them of how they really came to be. So we keep it a secret.

And therein lies the problem. Because then all it takes to initiate you into the halls of shame is for someone to sneer, 'Are you on your *period*?', saying period as though you'd just broken wind directly into their lunchbox, as though you had a heinous weakness to be ashamed of, as if you had an actual choice in the matter. Bit by bit, we learn that periods aren't something to be proud of. Our power isn't forgotten, but buried deeper. How can you defend yourself without pride in your body?

Most of us develop elaborate ways of communicating with our friends about periods. We use code words and meaningful eyebrow expressions that are met with knowing looks — anything to avoid saying the actual word.

To avoid being sprung, tampons and pads are slipped discreetly into sleeves before covert missions to the toilet. And if you really want to tend your bleeding vagina with complete stealth, you can even buy tampons with rustle-free packets so no one will ever hear the offensive and embarrassing sound of you having your period.

No wonder the mere word — *period* — can reduce girls to mortification; it wasn't even said on television until 1985 in a tampon ad with a spandex-clad Courtney Cox.

As a rule, ads for pads and tampons routinely featured a mysterious blue liquid, and exuberant girls dressed in white laughing as they participated in various sports. Meanwhile, in movies and sitcoms (written by men), the period served as a device for high drama. Finally, and more widely now, our bodies are being depicted and our stories are being told by women. But consider these poxy stereotypes (for the millionth time):

💜 When they are shown at all, periods are depicted as inherently gross, horrifying and tantamount to a crime scene. If a woman's filmic value hinges on her being sexy above all else, then menstruation renders her irrelevant. (Never mind that in real life menstruation can be an erotic, sensual experience.)

💜 While someone has a period they're portrayed as being overly emotional or even 'hysterical'. (If you want to dial your fury up several notches, do an online search to explore the history of 'female hysteria'.)

💜 To top it off, the bloody cherry on top of the pile of period-shame cake is the idea that during the time before your period arrives, when you are premenstrual, you are irrational at best and basically insane at worst.

💜 The worst thing about how periods are seen is that they *aren't*. They are invisible. How can you talk about something you can't see?

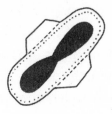

Unsurprisingly, as well as feeling shame about our physical periods, we learn to feel shame around the emotional aspects of the cycle because the only thing more offensive than menstrual blood is a woman with feelings, which is yet another thing that we can't talk about. The exception to this rule is that when you feel upset about something you should probably say to yourself dismissively, *Oh, it's nothing. It's just my hormones*, because *obviously* that's why we are overreacting. Right? Riiight. Never mind that Darryl was actually being a right asshole, and for once in the month you felt compelled to tell him. But instead, we are taught to silently chastise ourselves for not successfully maintaining the same emotional state (every single effing day) in spite of our changing hormones and varying abilities to put up with Darryl's shit. Once you get the hang of minimising your pesky feelings, it becomes second nature to doubt yourself and automatically assume blame. *Sorry, my fault. Sorry, just my hormones. Sorry. Sorry.* It's enough to make you feel crazy.

So we bleed in secret and learn the art of downplaying our feelings; we participate in the endurance test of pushing through being premenstrual and having periods like troopers month after month. Just imagine for a second what skill or attribute you could develop if you invested the same amount of energy into something else, *anything* else — oil painting, macramé or becoming an investment banker. We are relieved when the 'bad time' is over and we can finally do cartwheels in white jeans again, like we always wanted to. Yay. So far, so crap.

But now for the final crappy lesson in 'how to girl in a man's world', and it's a maths one: if being premenstrual and/or having my period makes me 'less than', or is something that I must push through (because obviously life is better during the other bits, right?), then that means for around half of my reproductively viable life, I am wishing it was over. Half. Of. My. Life — my actual life that I'm trying to actually just live.

As much as we try to maintain the virtually impossible facade of emotional and physical continuity all month long, inevitably we can't. This means we're set up to fail and to feel betrayed by our changing emotions, our bodies and, literally, *ourselves*. We become familiar with disappointment.

This is not good for us, obviously. But it turns out it is quite good for the many industries that are based upon this need to ignore, hide and disguise parts of our womanhood. There are endless solutions available, designed to convince you that you need fixing and improving. Designed to keep us out of the way. We pay and we pay and it never ends.

Is it any wonder, then, that we accept that there is nothing more to the menstrual cycle than making babies and avoiding periods at all costs?

The modern reality is that girls are more likely to grow up understanding the cycles on a washing machine or the dishwasher better than *their OWN cycle*!

HOW OTHER CULTURES 'GIRL'

We can learn so much from other cultures that knew — and still know — the importance of the menstrual cycle. There are many cultures for which a *menarche* or first period initiation celebration is a normal and important part of a girl's life.

Meet Tharanga — who shared her story during a workshop we ran together. She was born in Sri Lanka and remembers her first period celebration fondly, as though it was her 'little wedding'. She knew exactly what to expect, having seen older cousins go through it, and when she woke up with her period at twelve and her mother was out, her older sister put an iron knife under the bed to protect her, as was the custom. She was given new clothes to wear, and a big, beautiful coconut flower was placed in a clay pot next to her bed — a symbol that she was now ready to be a mother and also that she was never alone.

Tharanga was rarely alone during this time thanks to the many visitors who brought food (a tradition I think we'd all do well to subscribe to). While she rested and dreamed, a huge party was planned in her honour, and after seven days, she was taken into the garden for the ceremony. All the important women in her life were there. They helped her bathe and wash her hair for the first time since her bleeding began. Her aunties surrounded her underneath a jackfruit tree, and her mother poured water and flowers over her head. The jackfruit tree was cut ceremoniously so everyone could see the milk flowing, symbolising that Tharanga would one day also be able to make milk. She put her arms through a new yellow dress before being covered with a white scarf and taken to the front of her house.

At the door lay a big knife and a coconut, and before she could enter the party Tharanga had to chop the top off by herself. It was hard! But after all that resting she performed this test of strength successfully and drank the sweet juice. Then the party really began! All day long, relatives, neighbours and other villagers came in succession to celebrate her. The next day, happy and proud, she went to school and shared the leftover sweets from her party with her friends.

There are many variations on this rite of passage the world over, and the common themes include time alone, time with other women and elders, and various tests of strength and endurance followed by great celebration, feasts and dancing.

Sadly, the practising and passing on of many of these rituals (along with innumerable others) suffered due to colonisation. Of the menstrual traditions among Native Americans, Cutcha Risling Baldy writes in her book *We Are Dancing for You* that while 'it is impossible to deny the influence of the Western menstrual taboo on modern indigenous cultures and societies', these practices are intrinsic to decolonisation and the healing that must be done.

Baldy's book, and others like it, serves to restore cultural connections, undoing the damage caused by the outsiders who recounted these practices, even though they were unable to grasp the meaning of them. Baldy reminds us that stories about menstrual cycle rites were collected long ago by white men who were told about them by indigenous men who (understandably) may not have wanted those white ethnographers to know of their culture's most sacred practices. Many menstrual myths abound because the meaning of various rites and rituals was told to suit a narrative that placed white culture above indigenous cultures. So much of what we 'know' has been marred.

For example, it is frequently mentioned that Native American girls experiencing their first period 'are forbidden to touch food', which sounds like deprivation if you don't understand the reasons why. The why, as it turns out, is incredibly beautiful.

In a special series called 'Hidden World of Girls', broadcast in 2010 by *Morning Edition*, a show on America's National Public Radio (NPR),* Marla Bull Bear described the four-day coming-of-age ceremony her daughter took part in on the Yankton Sioux/Ihanktonwan Oyate Reservation in South Dakota. As she explained, the girls aren't allowed to touch any food during the ceremony because their mothers feed them, putting the food directly into their mouths. For these few days, during the bridge between being a girl and a woman, 'It's treating them like a baby one last time before they become women.' Of this bittersweet and important ritual, Marla Bull Bear said, 'No longer would she be my little girl to feed anymore. You really begin to start the foundation of what that adult relationship is with a mother and daughter.'

Monthly menstrual rituals are a way for women and girls from many cultures to come together for connection to their cycles and also, just as importantly, to each other. Again, this practice of being separated from the community has historically been portrayed negatively, but in fact, the isolation was to assist in them connecting more deeply to the power that came with menstruation. It was seen as a time of greater intuition that was *prized*.

*You can listen to this story here: www.npr.org/templates/story/story.php?storyid=129611281

HOW PERIODS (MIGHT HAVE) HAPPENED FOR EARLY HUMANS

Does menstruation make us human? To find out, let's rewind back about 300,000 years ago when our species (*Homo sapiens*) first emerged. One of the hallmarks of becoming human was a bigger brain, but the trade-off was that human babies were slower to develop and dependent for a longer period of time. Mothers needed more support, so they turned to the most reliable helpers: their own mothers.

Evolving human females also shared childcare burdens with their sisters — an arrangement that had practical and emotional benefits for both mothers and children. Eventually, women also persuaded the evolving primate male to offer reliable support with child rearing. But how?

One popular theory among anthropologists is proffered by Chris Knight in his book, *Blood Relations*. Knight's central premise is that our earliest symbolic cultural practices, including politics, art and religion, were organised around menstruation. My eyes widen as I type those words, but I really like them, and it makes sense.

Knight explains how, essentially, it was the females who likely created the taboo around menstruation — not because it was shameful, but because it could be used to establish the body as being sacred at this time. Females decided that they were tired of having to capitulate to one dominant boss (the biggest male), as their ape predecessors were forced to do. While their capacity to enjoy sex was at least as great as ours, the need to feed their children was greater. So, as a collective, the females decided that all of them would deny men sex in order to ensure that the males would provide enough food for the group.

When the moon was new and the nights were darkest, the women would gather together in dedicated spaces for a periodic (pun intended) 'sex strike'. Meanwhile, the men would gather and prepare for a big hunt that would take place during the build-up to the full moon — a time when it's easier to see large animals and not get eaten yourself. After the hunt, the men would return laden with provisions for the camp and be welcomed to commune with the women once more. In this way, the survival of the whole group was effectively ensured because of one simple, foundational principal: no meat = no sex.

Through regular time together, women's periods tended to synchronise. This is how menstrual blood came to be a signal that indicated this was not a time for sex, but for obtaining food. Sounds like a fair trade, doesn't it? Who hasn't had their period and thought, *Can't someone else get the food?*

Knight says that, over time, women created rituals and traditions around menstruation — including painting precious red ochre on themselves to symbolise bleeding. These practices enhanced the place of women in society and conveyed to the men that it was time to go hunting.

If Knight's hypotheses are correct, then somewhere along the way menstrual culture went awry. Knight's theory is that this began to happen in areas where large game animals became scarce. During the Ice Age, the capture of a mammoth meant that everyone had enough food to last a month. But as the Ice Age ended, conditions changed worldwide.

Only in Africa did very large game animals survive. Humans had to adjust to survive on smaller animals, and one monthly hunt was no longer sufficient to provide enough food. This changed everything.

Hunting practices were no longer regulated by the moon cycle, and so, for females, the self-imposed 'sex strikes' and women-only time fell by the wayside. As a result, they were less likely to bleed together and so collective blood (and ochre) as a signal was lost.

Knight explains that women lost their power once menstrual synchrony was no longer 'the basic ritual organising principal of social, sexual and economic life'. Spaces where women once came together to menstruate 'became male huts from which women were excluded, renamed as men's houses or temples'.

And that's not all: 'In many places, in order to prevent the whole system from collapsing, men started ritualising their own version of menstruation, by cutting their penises (or, in some places ears, noses, or arms) and bleeding together, shedding enormous amounts of blood.' Today, we know these practices as male circumcision, where the foreskin is cut.

Are you still with me? I know it's a lot, but get this: Knight ties a bow around these theories by pointing out that when men decided that their bloodletting rituals were more important, the familiar patterns of today's world religions came to the fore. 'Wherever you find these temples and churches, in Judaism, Christianity, they are men's huts writ large, male controlled and dominated.'

Knight suggests that these changes led to the prevalence of the patriarchal religious principles and male-dominated family and kinship practices characteristic of so much of the world today. In short, women were evicted from their sacred spaces and men 'faked' periods that were associated with power more than real periods. By making women and girls ashamed of menstruating, men were able to keep them away from the places where power was held and important decisions were made.

Menstrual stigma became one of the most powerful tools in history for keeping women down. It should come as no surprise that much of our 'his-story' features menstrual stigma. Remember who was doing the writing back then. The Bible, which has formed the basis for much of traditional Western culture, seems to be where period stigma was first recorded on paper some 2700 years ago along with the general theme that women were sent to help and obey men. From Leviticus 15: 'When a woman has a discharge . . . she shall be in her menstrual impurity for seven days, and whoever touches her shall be unclean until the evening.' It goes on to say that any thing or person that she touches will also be unclean, as will the person who touches the thing that she touches.

But maybe something was lost in translation? Maybe Leviticus was really saying, 'Hey, leave the bleeding ladies alone. They are busy bleeding and filth will reign upon you should you bother them! Serious, big time filth! Make them a sandwich, or else.'

Recently, after performing *My Greatest Period Ever*, a Muslim woman approached me to share a similar sentiment. She said that the premise of my whole show was actually supported by the Koran, which dates back 1400 years: 'Go apart from women during the monthly course, do not approach them until they are clean.' (The Koran, 2:222) She told me, 'Menstruation *was* seen as sacred, but the meaning has been lost.' People may view the temporary banishment from the kitchen or the temple as discriminatory, but it does make sense that menstruation is a time for women to be relieved of extra work and obligations and to accept support.

Around AD 77, a series of books called *Natural History* by a Roman called Pliny the Elder was published. This was the first Latin encyclopedia, and it was considered the authority on scientific matters until the Middle Ages. An extract from a passage on menstruation reads as follows: 'Contact with it [menstrual blood] turns new wine sour, crops touched by it become barren, grafts die, seeds in gardens are dried up, the fruit of trees fall off, the bright surface of mirrors in which it is merely reflected is dimmed, the edge of steel and the gleam of ivory are dulled, hives of bees die, even bronze and iron are at once seized by rust, and a horrible smell fills the air; to taste it drives dogs mad and infects their bites with an incurable poison.' You see? Whether people feared or respected them, periods have always held power. Obviously though, the fearmongers have had far too much airtime.

Whether or not you subscribe to Knight's theories, it's not difficult to see the power imbalance that still persists. Wherever there are positions of power, money and influence, there are fewer women — especially women on the margins of the mainstream. If you are a woman of colour hoping to improve or, indeed, just live your life, it's even harder to rise against the additional weight of cultural oppression.

SO WHERE DOES THAT LEAVE US?

It's a lot to compute, and it's hard to comprehend the impact that thousands of years of fake period news have had on us, both collectively and as individuals. Perhaps especially for you, dear reader. For you are a modern creature born at a time when (in theory, though not always in practice) women can go to university, have jobs, be the boss, have bank accounts, own houses, decide who (if anyone) they wish to marry and whether or not to have children (and if so, how many).

If you are reading this book now, you are one of the luckiest people in the world. Not just because this book is fabulous, if I do say so myself, but because you are educated and can read, and you or someone you know was wealthy enough to buy you a book in the first place. You have power. Maybe more than you know.

For that, we thank feminism and the many women and girls before us who had it bloody hard and fought (sometimes in small and quiet ways), over the last 100 years particularly, to win more equality. Some people scoff and say, 'So we don't need feminism anymore!' But we do. We're still a long way from equality. If you're unsure of where you stand on feminism, please take Caitlin Moran's simple test from her book *How to Be a Woman*: 'A) Do you have a vagina? And B) Do you want to be in charge of it? If you said "yes" to both, then congratulations, you are a feminist!' Her book contains more fantastic insights such as, 'I want a Zero Tolerance Policy on All the Patriarchal Bullshit.' Indeed, for that is exactly what menstrual stigma is — patriarchal bullshit — and it keeps women and girls from connecting deeply to themselves and to each other.

PERIOD POVERTY

Menstrual stigma also prevents people with periods from having what they need. This could mean pads, tampons or re-usable alternatives and somewhere to safely wash them — without judgment. It can mean access to a clean toilet and running water as well as menstrual education. These are all considered basic human rights, yet many are denied them.

And if girls don't have a safe place to change a pad (or a cloth) for fear of harassment, they are likely to miss out on school. Later in life they may not be afforded the opportunity to work, leading to them earning less money, being less independent and having less control over their own lives.

Chris Bobel, author of *The Managed Body*, cautions that the solution is more complicated than liberation through 'sanitary' pads. She reminds activists that, 'What a girl needs most is not products (or education about products), but to be freed from the menstrual mandate', the mandate being that periods are shameful.

No matter where you live, the root of period poverty is inextricably linked to menstrual stigma. But when women are empowered to create their own solutions, the benefits go beyond having something to bleed on. The Academy Award-winning documentary *Period. End of Sentence* tells the story of a group of Indian women from Kathikhera who began making and then marketing pads commercially — some earning money for the first time in their lives.

Not long ago, I met a woman who travels to Bougainville Island in Papua New Guinea a couple of times a year to teach women how to make their own re-usable pads. She told me that the women of that island sit on the beach or in the water and bleed into the sand for the duration of their periods when no other alternative is available to them. The women tell her that because of these pads they are now able to work and make money instead of sitting in the sand. They have a choice.

Being a Westerner doesn't confer immunity to this situation; if you're homeless or poor, you can find yourself having to choose between buying menstrual supplies or food for yourself and your children. This is especially true if you live in remote areas that are often under-resourced.

Have you ever gone without period products? Even just for a day or two? When I got my first period, I soon ran out of the complimentary pads from the plane toilet. I tried to wash and re-use them unsuccessfully. I spent the next few days using toilet paper, and I'd stash huge amounts of it in my pockets before leaving home in case the paper in the museums we visited turned out to be the waxy, thin, non-absorbent type. I had the ability to buy the supplies I needed but I was too embarrassed to speak about it.

There are many ways that people experience periods but what unites us all is a complete community buy-in says Bobel: 'To this end, everyone surrounding girls — boys, teachers, family members, religious leaders, policy makers, and so on — needs to challenge menstrual stigma. Girls need to be encircled in 360 degrees of body positivity.'

PERIOD SHAME

If I don't have what I need, I will likely experience more hardship during my period and then suffer more shame because of it. It's a vicious cycle. If I feel ashamed about my period, how can I possibly talk freely about my period *health* should I need to?

A UK survey by Plan International UK of 1004 girls aged fourteen to twenty-one showed exactly that:

💜 48% of the girls said they are embarrassed by their periods.

💜 79% of those with periods have been concerned by symptoms such as heavy bleeding, severe pain and irregularity.

💜 54% said they hadn't sought medical advice because they thought their symptoms were typical.

💜 27% said they were too embarrassed to speak to a health professional about their concerns while menstruating.

This is partly why conditions such as endometriosis can take so long to be diagnosed: girls endure excruciating pain and troubling symptoms but don't seek medical attention because of embarrassment and the feeling that they should 'put up with it'.

In a book called *About Bloody Time*, Karen Pickering and Jane Bennett document findings from a study of 3460 women and girls from Australia and 29 other countries:

💜 As many as 70% of girls aged between twelve and eighteen had negative feelings about their periods.

Of that 70%, 29% said that while there were some good things about their period, mostly it was bad, and 41% said they disliked everything about their period.

Periods can be painful and inconvenient, but women bear an additional burden when society treats periods with disdain. The reach of this internalised negativity can affect a whole life. If girls aren't encouraged to ask for, or feel unable to ask for, what they need when it comes to their bodies and period health, how can they feel equipped and entitled to voice their feelings and concerns about other things that are important to them? What else might they put up with because they feel they should? What might they not reach for because they feel they can't?

Of course, people have had positive period experiences, but traditionally, they have been the exception rather than the rule. Ask any older woman what having a period was like for her, or if she talked about it (or didn't). You'll see how these feelings are woven into our past, and how they still creep into our present.

Don't feel bad if you've ever felt bad about your period. No matter how progressive your parents were or are, the way we talk about something in the world can't help but impact the way we feel about that thing, especially if it happens to be part of us.

Shame is a barrier to pride. If you think you might be harbouring some shame, notice it, in whatever form it takes, and then treat it like a moth-eaten coat during a closet clear-out. We need to unpick these old threads so we can stop spending time and energy apologising for our bodies. Never, ever apologise for your period. Even to yourself.

WHEN IS THE BEST TIME TO INTRODUCE A CHILD TO PERIODS?

Now. Any time.

One day, when I was a fairly new mum, I was in the toilet with the door ajar. Then something happened that anyone with toddlers will relate to: I saw a small hand curl around the toilet door. I had my period at the time, and at that exact moment I happened to be removing a tampon (this is before I knew that re-usable products existed).

My instinct was to gently steer him out of the toilet with my foot. *Out you hop.* I thought. But I'd been working as a sexual health educator for a while by then, and my logical mind took over just before his face popped into view. He surveyed the scene — my tampon literally mid-air — and met my eyes.

'Hi, Mum,' he said sweetly.

'Hello,' I replied.

He craned his neck around the door to see what I was holding. 'Mum, what are you doing?'

I took a deep breath. 'Well, remember how I told you about how I bleed every month? This is a tampon and it's one of the ways that I catch the blood.'

'Oh,' followed by silence, and then, 'Mum, can I see it?'

'What? My tampon?'

At this point I really did not want to be having this conversation. I wanted to exit the toilet in an expedient fashion. But his innocent little face was so curious, inquisitive and loving that I softened my face, too: 'Oh, okay. Sure.'

He smiled, stepped through the toilet door and then had a close look at the tampon I was holding.

I waited patiently for it to be over. But what he said next made me realise why this little chat was so powerful.

'Mum . . . is that . . . gross?'

Now don't get me wrong, a used tampon may not be your idea of beauty, but did I want this little boy to associate periods with something gross? I saw his face reading mine, searching to see how he should understand this thing that happens to his mother, who he loves (and, indeed, to half of the population). I realised that what my face said in that moment and the words that I chose were incredibly important — they would inform his understanding and appreciation of women and their bodies.

I looked right into his eyes and said, 'No darling. It's actually amazing, this blood. It comes from inside of my body where every month I make a brand-new nest and, if I want to, I can grow a baby in there — in my actual body.' I pointed to my womb.

His eyes widened and then his face cracked into an incredulous smile. 'Mum! Thath tho cool!' (He had a lisp at the time.)

I smiled back at him. 'Yes, darling, it is very cool. Now will you hop out please?'

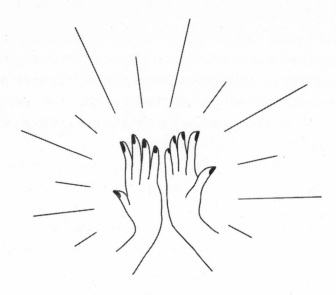

PERIOD POSITIVITY

If menstrual taboo is at the very heart of patriarchy and female oppression, then period positivity is where the antidote lies. We need to support all women and girls living all kinds of lives to shake off as much oppression as humanly possibly in our own lifetime. We do this by banding together and supporting each other using every little bit of power we have. Trust me when I say you have this power in spades — it's in your pants! Your period powers.

Unless you've been living under a rock you'll know that periods are #trending thanks to menstrual activism, art, celebration, gender equality work and certain dipstick politicians who give us good reasons to rally. The moment has evolved into a full-blown movement, and the tidal wave of crimson is undeniable.

Not everyone will choose to make a song and dance about it (hello!); you many not choose to run the London Marathon while free-bleeding (as artist Kiran Gandhi did) or paint protest portraits of politicians with period blood (as artist Sarah Levy did). But change is coming, and we are starting to see what it looks like when the power of women is fully realised.

At the time of writing this book, there have been countless other books published about periods. There are new apps to help you sync your work-outs to your cycle, and a documentary about periods has won an Oscar. In the southern Indian state of Kerala, up to five million women joined hands to make a 'women's wall', to challenge a religious custom that precluded women of menstruating age from entering the Sabarimala Temple, one of the most visited temples in the world. On the other side of the road, men lined up to show their support.

Women the world over are rising up and elevating the menstrual taboo to period pride. And this pride is connecting us all to ourselves, to other women and even to the planet as many bleeders come to grips with the impact of menstruation on the environment. All the plastic applicators washed up on our beaches, and all the pads and tampons wrapped in plastic, every one of those non-biodegradable items will lie in landfill for hundreds of years. So every time you choose a more sustainable option — whether that's bleeding into your period pants or pouring the blood from your menstrual cup — you are changing the world one drop at a time. Less waste, more pride.

When you see your blood as the proof of your power, you become your own sacred temple. Della Rae Morrison is an Aboriginal actor, songwriter and activist of the Bibulman Noongar people in Western Australia. She told me about a time when she was on tour, passing through Warburton after driving for hours. With desert all around her, she pulled over for a bush wee and to stretch her tired legs. 'It was sunsetting, the big sky was luminous bright blue with an amazing orange sun.' She crouched behind the long, dry spinifex and then looked down. 'My blood was bright red on the red dirt. Euphoria went through my body and I savoured the feeling. I wanted to cry out but I just smiled to myself.'

My most ardent wish is that every girl grows up not only equipped physically in a culture that has normalised menstruation but also knowing that she has an ally in her body that will give her strength, guidance and solace. Then, a generation of girls can understand and use the gifts of their cycle instead of fighting the very forces that drive them.

If you are reading this and feel fecked off that you are no longer a girl who could have used this information, I feel you. So much. There's a grief to realising that your body and soul have been the target of toxic patriarchal paradigms. I hope you can meet this with softness and find strength in it, too. And if, after purging yourself of shame, you discover that there is still some anger about all of this, use it. We need to keep stoking the fires of change until all menstruators can bleed in peace.

I don't want to pass this rubbish on to a daughter of mine or anyone else's. It's time to burn that ugly old coat and plant in its place so deep and so safe a proud strength that we are reminded of every month: powers that we treasure and pass on to our daughters.

This book has been written to help you do that, and to help you help those who'll come after you. It will guide you as you learn about these powers and how to love yourself best all month long. If we want women, girls and menstruators at the front, ruling the world or doing whatever the hell they want, we need to meet our power and to practise it, one period at a time. You'll have around 450 of them in your lifetime, so you may as well use them!

And now, welcome to your womb.

CHAPTER 2

A CRASH COURSE iN LADY SCiENCE

There is basic biology information in this section that you may be aware of, but it can be useful to hear things in a different way.

Your first period shows up anywhere between the ages of nine and fifteen (twelve/thirteen are the average). Just as when you were a newborn baby getting to know your body, it can take some adjusting and time to grow into your new menstruating self.

Imagine a butterfly about to burst from its chrysalis: while it writhes around inside, its wings are strengthening in preparation for flight. Similarly, our bodies and cycles can feel bound up and unsteady while becoming accustomed to new levels of hormones. But with every cycle, your body refines her response. In her excellent book *Period Repair Manual*, Dr Lara Briden explains that it can take up to twelve years to establish a regular, healthy menstrual cycle as your hormones slowly but surely 'carve out rivers'.

YOUR WOMB

It seems only fitting that we begin our tutelage with a visit to the womb, also known as a uterus. I love the word 'womb'. Phonetically, it's a combination of 'woman' and 'room' — beginning with a whisper and ending with a hum: *womb*.

What a mysterious place, where one day we might grow a human. Does this ever stop being mind-blowing? That we can GROW PEOPLE INSIDE OF US? No, it doesn't. Even if we never do it, it's a pretty powerful possibility to just walk around with. We are custodians of life, all kinds of life, and this is where we hold it.

To fully appreciate its power, 'feel in' to your womb, where there is space for whatever it is that you want to give life to. For a sense of its size and shape, make a fist and place it just above your pubic bone, between your hips, nice and low. This is where it is. It's connected to your vagina by your cervix, which acts as a portal that literally anchors your womb within your body.

Every single month (or thereabouts), your womb uses tissue and fresh blood cells to make a thick, luxurious lining. This is like a nest within its innermost layer, the *endometrium*. Once it becomes clear that you will not be making a human that month, your womb, in all its wisdom, lets go. And so begins your period.

The muscles of your *myometrium*, the thick middle layer of the womb, contract to remove all traces of the 'nest'. If it feels like you're being squeezed in all directions, you are! With muscles that run top to bottom, in figure eights and in rings around your womb, you might sometimes wish they wouldn't have to try quite so hard, but bear in mind, they are also using the opportunity to practise for a potential future labour.

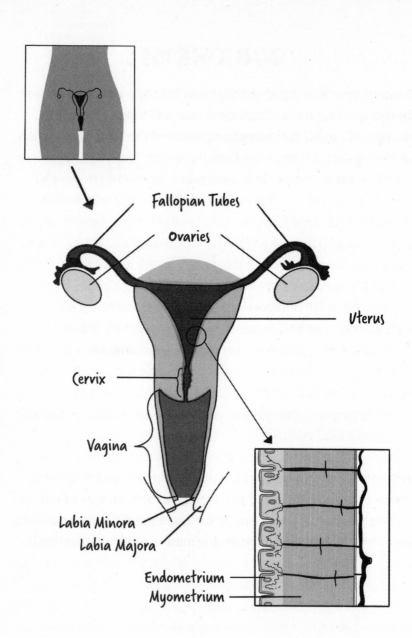

Fallopian Tubes

Ovaries

Uterus

Cervix

Vagina

Labia Minora

Labia Majora

Endometrium

Myometrium

YOUR OVARIES

So much attention is paid to the bleeding part, you'd be forgiven for thinking that a menstrual cycle was just the presence or absence of blood, but the real superstar of the cycle is ovulation. Without it we wouldn't even have hormones. You've got a couple of purses full of pearls hidden deep in your pelvis, one on either side of your womb, packed with immature egg cells, known as *oocytes*. Think of your mother, inside of her mother: by the time she was as big as a mango, stretching and wriggling around in a warm salty ocean, she had two tiny ovaries filled with all of the eggs she would ever have. While you were a little star in her sky, for a time, all three generations were together. Your grandmother's body is the land where your life first took root.

The ovaries, our primary reproductive organs, are in constant communication with the pituitary gland (a pea-sized part of our brain), carving out our rivers to make sure everything is just right. If it is, a mature egg is released every month. This conversation is what gives you your cycle.

It turns out women and men are more similar than not, and many of our supposed differences can be attributed to gender stereotypes that come into play from the moment we're born (sometimes before). However, a fundamental difference between women and those born biologically male is our menstrual cycle.

IF YOU ARE BIOLOGICALLY MALE

The same type of human tissue that makes up ovaries is used in utero to configure testicles, which are just as important. Testicles produce testosterone, the major hormonal driver in men, and men have a cycle, too. Although there is some fluctuation, the hormonal 'river' of testosterone is fairly constant, and the cycle runs its course over just one day.

Testosterone levels are highest in the morning (as is sexual desire and the ability to focus), and they drop slightly as the day goes on, which is why group work can be more effective in the afternoon once a bit of the *get out of my way, I have things to do* drive has worn off. Levels are lowest at night (often making this the best time for difficult conversations), and they are replenished during sleep.

Although things are certainly changing, it is still true that if you are a man in the world with a man's hormones, you can pretty much walk out of your house and feel like the world is set up just for you. Because it is.

You can walk into an air-conditioned building and feel normal because thermostats are set to the average comfortable temperature — for men. And if you take a new medicine, you can rest assured that it's been tested — on men. Until recently, drug trials were *only* done on men because men were considered the biological norm. Women were treated as hormonal anomalies and simply prescribed smaller doses, as if they were 'small men'. And this was problematic because, as we now know, women respond differently to diseases as well as the medications necessary to treat them.

And yet this difference in how we cycle is largely unknown. As a result, we are all — male, female and non-binary — obliged to adhere to a male cycle. With no room or appreciation for deviation, we are expected *to be the same*. Every. Single. Day.

IF YOU ARE BIOLOGICALLY FEMALE

Women don't have just one way of being that fades in intensity over the course of a day and renews every morning. We are ruled not by the sun, but by the moon. Our cycle runs over a whole month, and within each cycle there are two major hormonal events: ovulation and menstruation. You are always either experiencing or preparing for one of these two happenings. Thus, throughout the month, you have four ways of *being* (aka the cyclical superpowers).

It's not that weird that this isn't common knowledge because, as we already know, men have been at the helm of the very important things, and understanding periods and cycles just wasn't seen as that important (for them at least). This is the real reason why people think female hormones are 'crazy' or 'complicated': they actually just have no idea. The true complication comes from having to act as if we don't have female hormones when we do. To revisit the river analogy, this means that instead of going with the flow, we must swim upstream. If we don't do this, we might be labelled irrational, unpredictable, too emotional, too sensitive, too much.

Some people will feel uneasy about this conversation. They worry that by openly acknowledging how our changing female hormones can affect our energy levels and emotions, we will be made vulnerable to being reduced to our biology and its perceived limitations. Indeed, it's happened before, and it was no mean feat to get as far as we have in terms of equality. So much work has been done by feminists to prove that women are equal, competent and deserving of the corner office and the top job or whatever it is that they strive for; but the victory is a bittersweet one if being considered equal to a man means you have to act like one.

Although being a (white) male has historically been considered the default setting, from a biological perspective, it's actually the other way around. Until about six weeks of gestation, we all begin life as female. According to Charles Darwin, this primordial female nature harks back to the effects that the lunar tides had on early life forms for the first two-and-a-half billion years. Single-celled organisms floated and reproduced asexually in a layer of salty fluid that covered the earth's surface like a womb. He believed that the menstrual cycle was originally inspired by this lunar tidal effect and that this is why menstrual cycles and lunar cycles are of a very similar length. So strong was his conviction, Darwin even postulated that the prostate gland might have been a rudimentary uterus.

Billions of years after life began, we are still learning of our nature. Male and female cycles are exquisitely different. Not better than the other, but different. It's just that male cycles have had the megaphone for much of our known 'his-story'. In light of this and in the absence of true representation, it's time to celebrate the daylights out of/into our cycles. Your cycle is the motherland of your superpowers.

THE MENSTRUAL CYCLE IN TWO HALVES

To start with, let's look at the menstrual cycle and the hormones that drive it. Within the one cycle are two phases: the *follicular* and the *luteal*.

The *follicular phase* begins on the first day of menstruation (bleeding) at the beginning of your cycle. It's called the follicular phase because the focus is not on the bleeding at all but on the maturing follicles (the eggs) within your ovaries. Your body is built to simultaneously bleed and move on towards the next egg to be released, letting go but still reaching towards new potential. You begin this first half of your cycle with a hormonal hibernation, before you unfurl and expand, physically and energetically, as you move towards the peak of your fullness at ovulation.

The *luteal phase* begins once your egg has been released. Your extremely clever ovary makes a little temporary gland from the space where the egg was, like a little shrine of remembrance. This gland is called the *corpus luteum* (which is just Latin for 'yellow body'), hence the name, and it produces the crucially important hormone progesterone. When the luteal phase begins, you are on top of the metaphoric world, fuelled by your unbridled potential, which you use in all manner of ways until it's gone. As you prepare to cross back over into the follicular phase again, your next period arrives once progesterone and oestrogen levels have finished dropping.

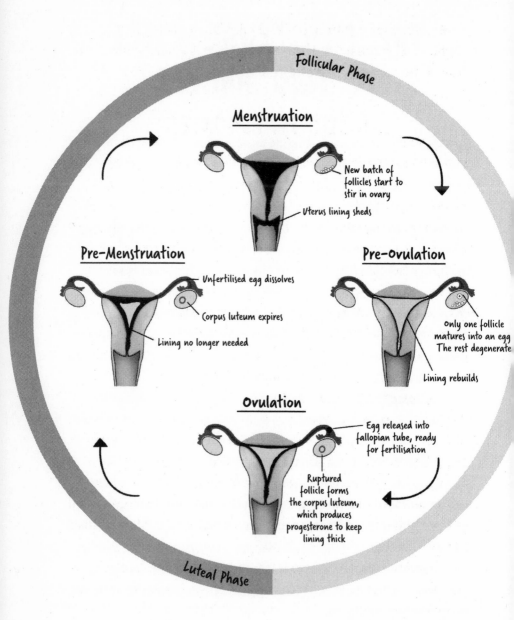

Follicular Phase

Menstruation

New batch of follicles start to stir in ovary

Uterus lining sheds

Pre-Menstruation

Unfertilised egg dissolves

Corpus luteum expires

Lining no longer needed

Pre-Ovulation

Only one follicle matures into an egg The rest degenerate

Lining rebuilds

Ovulation

Egg released into fallopian tube, ready for fertilisation

Ruptured follicle forms the corpus luteum, which produces progesterone to keep lining thick

Luteal Phase

Expansion and contraction. Just like the moon becoming brighter and more powerful before receding into complete darkness. Always moving and always changing. Cycling.

LADY HORMONES

Now it's time to take a tour through the cycle and meet each hormone in its own right. Introducing (drum roll, please) the main players (not in order of appearance):

Oestrogen: Evolutionary biologists tell us that oestrogen was the first-ever hormone to evolve. It's what ultimately makes us into women. It's stored in our fat cells and gives us our lovely shapes, readying our bodies to create life (as *well* as art, music, ideas and other things) and sustain it. In the first half of the cycle, oestrogen is the alpha, the lady boss fuelling everything you create with your mind, body, heart and hands, along with two supporting co-stars, follicular stimulating hormone and luteinising hormone, and a lick of . . .

Testosterone: *Not* just for men. While we don't have as much as they do (we'd probably combust if we suddenly did), we're more sensitive to it, so pound for pound what we do have is pretty potent. It's here for a good time, not a long time, but it's instrumental to maintaining our overall health and energy as well as bone and muscle strength and our sexual desire. After all that, it's time to meet . . .

Progesterone: Ahhh, progesterone. Known as nature's feel-good hormone, it has a calming effect as it smooths over all the excitement of ovulation like an antidote to balance out the effects of oestrogen. Progesterone gives our bodies a chance to drop into the easy lane. It's hard to illustrate progesterone levels in the graph on page 63 because we have SO much of it. At peak production, we have around 100 times more progesterone than we do oestrogen.

After millions of years of evolution, our whole bodies are geared to respond to progesterone. Without it, we're in trouble. With every single ovulation, you produce this beneficial hormone that has a protective effect on your body in the short and the long term. Dr Lara Briden, author of *Period Repair Manual*, likens it to a monthly investment in our future health. Like a peaceful ruler in a kaftan, progesterone swans in to govern the after party/last half of the cycle with a gentle hand and a block of chocolate.

LADY HORMONES IN ACTION: THE FOLLICULAR PHASE

First, I should say that the given figures for each phase length are averages — one size does not fit all. To see how your cycle might work over your own four phases, peruse the table on page 74.

MENSTRUATION: DAY 1 (THE FIRST DAY OF BLEEDING)

Most of us will bleed for about 5 days, but a few more or a few less is also normal. Behind the bleeding scenes, our faithful friend the pituitary gland readies itself to pump out . . .

Follicular stimulating hormone (FSH): This hormone has two major moments, or peaks. The first occurs once you are menstruating in full swing: your pituitary sends FSH from your brain to your ovaries, and a batch of new eggs wriggles with anticipation. They begin to stir.

PRE-OVULATION: DAY 6(ISH) (AFTER YOU STOP BLEEDING)

This phase lasts from the end of your bleed until ovulation at around Day 14, or later if your cycle is longer than 28 days (the longer your cycle, the later you ovulate). The champion hormone of this stage is . . .

Oestrogen: *(narrated as a horseracing commentator)* This hormone starts ramping up towards the end of your period. While the follicles in your ovaries get busy guzzling up the FSH, they grow bigger and more luscious and start their own pro-duction line. In fact, they start making oestrogen in a sort of hormonal mutual appreciation society with the pituitary. By the time your period finishes, the chosen follicle has reached about half its full size, which is no small thing; at full size, the egg is the largest human cell — large enough to see with the human eye. As the follicles grow, they produce more and more oestrogen. They are *pumped*, quite literally, and so are you; it's as if they're preparing for a big race (which they are: ovulation). Once oestro-gen peaks, the red flag unfurls as a signal to your body that you are ready to release one precious egg. To help with ovulation, your pituitary sends in . . .

Luteinising hormone (LH): The peak in oestrogen serves as a love letter to the pituitary gland, telling it that the body is indeed ready for LH to join the party in a big way. And it does this gladly with a massive spike, which plays a critical role in prompting the most mature egg in the ovary to make its grand debut.

More FSH: With the massive LH surge, FSH re-emerges for its dramatic second spike. Together, LH and FSH encourage the egg to take the plunge and leave the ovary. The deal is sealed with ...

Testosterone: The peak in testosterone gives the important final nudge before ovulation. When testosterone peaks just before ovulation, you can feel more driven, inclined to take risks and even euphoric and superhuman. You ARE a super human.

This hormonal combination culminates in ovulation, marking the end of the follicular phase. And now we make party!

LADY HORMONES IN ACTION: THE LUTEAL PHASE

This part of the cycle is about being ready for greatness: a baby, a new invention, nailing a driving test . . . the choice is yours.

POST OVULATION: DAY 14(ISH) TO DAY 20(ISH)

Following ovulation, the egg has left the follicle and the body is priming itself for a potential pregnancy, and to that end, we are flooded with . . .

Progesterone: After we ovulate, the ruptured follicle forms the *corpus luteum* and produces progesterone like it's going out of fashion. Why? In case its previous tenant, the egg, gets lucky, meets a sperm and manages to make it to the womb. This little golden gland provides enough progesterone to maintain the lining of the womb *just in case* the egg is fertilised. As the name suggests (*pro gest*, from *gestation*), progesterone promotes gestation, or pregnancy.

As progesterone begins to climb, oestrogen makes a second appearance, and together they soar as though anything is possible until you are . . .

PREMENSTRUAL: DAY 21 TO DAY 28, OR THEREABOUTS

Having these hormones (namely progesterone and oestrogen) is what sustains the lovely nest in your womb. As soon as your body gets wise to the fact that you won't be sponsoring the little egg to fruition, your hormones drop — suddenly. Over a few days, they decline exponentially until they are gone like the last autumn leaf. Without them, your womb knows to let go.

And then you begin again.

The pituitary and the ovaries produce this whole team of hormones, fuelling cycle after cycle. Like two best friends having a sleepover, they chat nonstop, or at least until menopause. By this time, they hardly need to say another (hormonal) word; they've heard each other's stories so often, they know them by heart. After hundreds of these cycles, you will know yourself by heart, too, and won't need to bleed to be reminded; you will *become* your power. But first you must practise it, and you will, with every cycle, and every phase within it.

And THIS is where your superpowers finally come in.

CHAPTER 3

INTRODUCING YOUR SUPERPOWERS
(THE GIST)

It's time to move on from the science of your cycle to the artistry of it. It's the difference between knowing something and *feeling* it, and knowing that you feel that way for a reason. This is where you find the jewels in the crown. Welcome to your superpowers.

The graph opposite doesn't just show how your main hormone levels change; it's also a map for the four phases of the menstrual cycle — Dream, Do, Give and Take. (This chart depicts an average cycle of 28 days, but if you have a shorter or longer cycle, then the table on page 74 will help you figure out how long your phases might be.) Notice the mountains and the valleys, and how they correspond to ovulation and menstruation. Here's how it works.

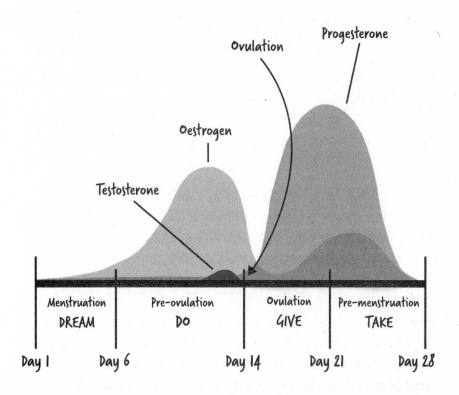

TIME TO DREAM (MENSTRUATION)

After making it down the mountain that was your last month, your hormones flatline. You're ready to let go and menstruate. It's time to find a quiet cave in a peaceful valley and stop, drop and feel. If possible, surrender to the slowness and stillness that your body craves. Fill your cup to the brim with self-love — the more energy you conserve now, the more you'll have for the month ahead. Dial in to your intuition and ponder big questions:

💜 How do I feel about the month I've just had?

💜 What will I grow and give life to next?

You have the gentle power to **dream** deeply now, about new ideas, inspiration, solutions, projects; everything is ahead of you but it all starts here, at your beginning.

TIME TO DO (PRE-OVULATION)

After you finish bleeding, your oestrogen rises until you're ready to skip on out of that cave like nobody's business. You emerge resplendent, restored, recharged and ready to climb up that huge mountain. Whatever it takes, you can **do** it. As you ready yourself to drop a new golden egg, this is your power week.

After the lovely hibernation of the Dream phase, it can be a bit overwhelming to step out and up with this surge within you. Just put one foot in front of the other and get started. Whatever 'it' is, you've got the power to do it.

TIME TO GIVE (POST-OVULATION)

You champion! You made it to the top of the mountain. At ovulation, take a moment (or better yet, a few days) to marvel and to revel in all of this beauty. It's everywhere — around you, IN you, all over you! What a thing to be alive. You have a bounty of hormones after ovulation and this abundance can make you feel like saying yes! Yes! To everything! Everyone's invited to celebrate how fabulous you are as you **give** this playful and exuberant energy back into the world around you. Everything is possible, until suddenly it isn't.

TIME TO TAKE (PRE-MENSTRUATION)

Your hormonal cup is fast emptying, and there's just enough left to get you back down the mountain. Look behind you and reflect on how far you've come this month; you have dreamed, done and given your absolute all and it was wonderful, but now you must prepare to let go again. After saying 'Yes!' last week with such generosity, you might find yourself saying 'Hell, NO!' now with a touch of protective ferocity. There is an intensifying need to turn your back on the world and connect to your deepest self while you make your way down.

Go at your own pace. Your potent superpower now is to **take,** to take the goodness from this whole cycle, and whatever else you need (the last piece of cake, the comfiest chair, your sweet time), to get ready to bleed. You are bound for the valley again.

A HEADS-UP ON THE BiG FEELiNGS

During Do (pre-ovulation) and Give (post-ovulation), it's generally easier to be kinder to yourself because these middle two phases are more socially acceptable (because you're *doing and giving*, duh). Others reward us more during these phases, too, and that feels pretty good.

Generally, if we feel good, we don't question it, we just feel good. How lovely to feel strong, capable, positive, at ease, excited, sociable and confident. But, unless you are a very rare breed of unicorn, you absolutely won't feel like this all of the time. You'll climb some incredible mountains (metaphorically speaking), and you'll feel on top of the world and have all kinds of adventures up there. But, dear woman, when the time comes, you gotta come back down.

It will come as no surprise that the other half of the cycle — Take (pre-menstruation) and Dream (menstruation) — can present more challenges. When we feel overwhelmed, tired, grumpy, irritable, impatient, frustrated or 'peopled out', we can turn these feelings inwards, against our precious selves, and be inclined to think the problem is with us. Many people wish they could skip these less socially acceptable parts of the cycle altogether (which is why you'll notice that the Dream and Take chapters are a little longer, with more strategies to help you navigate them). It's important to remind ourselves that the real problem is feeling you are meant to be the same all month long when you aren't.

Back when I didn't really understand my menstrual cycle or how it affected me, I used to hear the phrase, 'What goes up must come down' and take it as an affront. *It does not!* I would think, with indignation. *How negative!* I insisted to myself that everything could be wonderful all of the time if only I could just be positive. I felt this way partly because I had quite a good life and partly because I'm a natural optimist, but mostly because the world is hooked on this idea that we must always be productive, happy, useful, efficient and living our best lives. It took me years of exploring my own cycle and getting to know it inside out before I stopped fearing and resisting the coming down part, and stopped feeling guilty for not being able to keep the wonderfulness up.

In time, you'll find (hopefully sooner than I did) that the more introspective phases (Take and Dream) can be beautiful; not only that, but it's also entirely necessary to surrender to them in order to garner the stamina required to make the most of the more outward-looking phases (Do and Give).

The alternative — powering through life regardless of phase — is unsustainable. That kind of living will not make you a well and happy individual, regardless of whether you've a cycle or not. Constantly forging ahead at great heights, exposed to the elements, with the wind rushing in your ears and no time to rest is a recipe for disaster. Your body will ache as it whispers hopefully, 'Will you rest soon?' It's quite normal and understandable to feel less tolerant of people around you when you are premenstrual, just as it's quite normal to feel more tired of normal life when you have your period.

There are lots of ways that cycles present, and the way they make us feel varies from person to person, but one example I'll touch on is premenstrual dysphoric disorder (PMDD), which dishes out the biggest of the big feelings for around one in twenty women whose bodies respond to progesterone differently. At the point of ovulation, instead of that hormone having a calming effect, it causes extreme anxiety, depression and irritability. For those with PMDD, the path to cycle superpowers can be paved with natural disasters.

A friend of mine, Karen Lee, said, 'It's like a cyclone you know is coming for you every month. Everything is dark when you're inside it, and it can feel like you have to spend the rest of the month repairing the damage. Oh, and you're the cyclone.' Instead of feeling the urge to Give, it can feel more like *Mother of god, give me a forking break.* If PMS is a time for reckoning, perhaps women with PMDD are carrying the mother lode. More research, support and undersatnding is needed for sufferers. (For more about PMDD, visit the International Association for Premenstrual Disorders at iapmd.org.)

Whatever emotions you're experiencing, listen and make adjustments where you can. By seeing yourself through the lens of your menstrual cycle, you'll come to realise that at different times of the month you just have different needs and different gifts. Women aren't straight lines; we move like waves.

HOW TO TRACK YOUR CYCLE

There's no wrong or right way to track your cycle, just start on any day you like and aim to continue for at least three months. Use this book as a companion, and read others like it to deepen your understanding of your body and your cycle (there's a list of great resources on page 267). Talk to your body. Listen to it. What is it that you need? Quiet time alone? To be barefoot in nature? A good chat with a friend? How do you feel physically and emotionally? What helps and what doesn't on each day? Write it all down.

You'll soon get a pretty good picture of how your body works, and you'll start to see patterns. Once you get to know your phases, you'll know what to expect and consequently there will be fewer surprises, better ways to prepare and care for yourself, and better ways to be. Eventually, you will be an expert in you.

If you want to really understand your body and become savvier about the phase transitions, you can also track physical symptoms such as your cervical fluid (more on that later), period flow, body temperature (more on that later, too) and even the position of your cervix. These are all valuable signs to help you figure out where you are in your cycle. And, in the event that you require a doctor's advice at some point, this information will be useful. But the most important thing to monitor is how you feel. If you've never tracked your cycle before, you are a mere three months from being a period queen. Your crown awaits!

TOP TRACKING TIPS

❤ Take your time and enjoy it, like you would getting to know a new friend.

❤ Begin by tracking your bleeding so you know when your period is due. Day 1 is when it starts.

❤ Find out when you ovulate. Ovulation is the most important part of your cycle. Generally it occurs 14 days before your next period starts.

❤ Treat yourself to a nice new journal. Make tracking into a daily ritual. Cup of tea? Light a candle?

❤ Every night, jot down what day you are on and how you feel. What were your moods, energy levels, anything that's important to you. What did you feel drawn to focus on? What was easy and what was hard? What helped?

❤ Write a few lines or draw a picture.

❤ If you stop for a while, just start again when you remember.

❤ Consider using an app once you've got the hang of tracking how you feel. Include the physical changes of each phase.

❤ Invite your friends to join you in tracking their cycles.

❤ Look up, like millions of women before you, to notice the moon. Maybe you'll be reminded of your cycle when you notice hers.

USE YOUR SUPERPOWERS BY PLANNING FOR THEM

By writing down what you need and referring to it, you show your body that you are listening, that it matters and that you will remember what worked well for it in the months ahead. Listen to what your body is telling you, then respond accordingly and you'll be rewarded. It's that simple, and this is when your superpowers really come into play.

As you continue to observe your cycle, you will learn about your physical and emotional landscapes in more detail, and see how they affect each other. Soon, you'll be able to predict upcoming changes. Once you can do that, you'll be able to plan for them. I know scriptwriters, students, mums, scientists, painters and popstars who swear by planning around their cycles.

Knowing where you'll be in your cycle will help you make decisions. Whether it's tackling big projects, important social events, difficult situations or deciding whether you want to go camping on that particular weekend with those particular people at a location that requires a five-hour drive while sitting next to a dog. This is how you scaffold, so that you know when to push and when to pull (the pin, if necessary).

💜 Try highlighting sections of your diary with four different colours to reflect your (predicted) phases and remind you what tasks will be easiest for you, and when.

💜 If work allows, plan weekly tasks according to your phases.

- Pay attention to clues over time. Do you always feel energetic on Day 6 or do you sometimes feel wobbly? What made you feel that way? Did you do something differently that time?

- Once you understand what makes some days harder, avoid these tasks/activities/people on those days next month.

- Maximise the easy days. You'll start to get a picture of exactly how you would like to spend them in future cycles.

- Set intentions as you transition into each phase for how you want to care for yourself. What you want to focus on? How do you want to use your superpower?

- Notice where you feel most at home in your cycle and which phases are more challenging.

- Delve deep and focus on one particular phase per cycle to learn about your nuances and strengths. Finetune your superpowers one by one to discover your brilliance.

- Divide your wardrobe into phases: comfy clothes for Dream, activewear for Do, fancy for Give and dramatic for Take.

- Condense your findings after three months into a cheat sheet with tips and self-care recipes for each phase. Print this and keep it by your desk, stick it in your diary or save a photo of it to your favourites and update it often.

- If an issue feels Really Big? Run it through a whole cycle. Check in to see how you're feeling about it every few days to taste how it feels over a month.

- Ponder this personal data to maximise your cycle, your month and your WHOLE LIFE.

ANY QUESTIONS?

When you travel the world doing a show about periods, you talk to lots of people about them. And you tend to be asked a few of the same questions. Here are some I am frequently asked.

HOW LONG IS MY CYCLE MEANT TO BE?

Just like with every other physical thing — the shape of your nose, the length of your fingers, your resting heart rate — we are all a little different. The average cycle is 28 days, which takes into account all of the shorter/longer cycles that people have. Anything between 21 and 35 days is considered normal.*

When you first start to have a cycle, you can have long ones of up to 45 days while your body gets the hang of ovulating — this is completely normal. With every ovulation, your period should arrive around two weeks later, and once you ovulate regularly, your period should become regular, too. Assuming you are ovulating and have a relatively healthy cycle, it can always be divided into four phases (no matter how long your cycle is). Remember, the first day of your period (bleeding) is the first day of your cycle. The day before your next period is the last day of your cycle.

WHAT IF I'M ON THE PILL (OR ANY OTHER HORMONAL CONTRACEPTION)?

I'll talk about this more on page 117, but the short answer is anything that stops you from ovulating will prevent you from making

*In a study with 120,000 women using a tracking app, 65 per cent of their cycles were between 25 and 30 days; there is a wide range of 'normal'.

Cycle lengths and the four phases

Average cycle length in days	Dream	Do	Give	Take
36	1–5	6–21	22–28	29–36
35	1–5	6–20	21–27	28–35
34	1–5	6–19	20–26	27–34
33	1–5	6–18	19–25	26–33
32	1–5	6–17	18–24	25–32
31	1–5	6–16	17–23	24–31
30	1–5	6–15	16–22	23–30
29	1–5	6–14	15–21	22–29
28	1–5	6–13	14–20	21–28
27	1–5	6–12	13–19	20–27
26	1–5	6–11	12–18	19–26
25	1–5	6–10	11–17	18–25
24	1–5	6–9	10–16	17–24
23	1–5	6–8	9–15	16–23
22	1–5	6–7	8–14	15–22

your own hormones.* The other very important point is that the pill does NOT regulate periods. You may still notice your phases, but without *your* hormones, your cycle won't be the same.

HOW DO YOU DETERMINE WHICH PHASE YOU ARE IN?

I'll go into more detail about how to notice the physical transition signs within these phases in Chapters 4–7.

HOW LONG WILL EACH PHASE LAST FOR?

Based on an average cycle of 28 days, we know the luteal phase (the last half of the cycle) is always about 14 days long, no matter how long the entire cycle is. If you have a longer cycle, this means your follicular phase (the first half of your cycle) is longer, too. Therefore the phase with the most flexibility is the Do (or pre-ovulatory) phase. (See the chart opposite.)

You might be someone who cycles like clockwork every month and can plan months in advance, or you might be more like me: I have a variable 28–31-day cycle, so I estimate the phases in my diary based on that, and then tweak as needed. I take my temperature to know when I've ovulated (and when to predict future ovulations), and this means I can also assume my period will arrive about two weeks later. Another sign that your period is close is that your temperature will drop a day or two before it's due. Sometimes your cycle won't flow as predicted. The most common reason for this is stress.

*The hormonal IUD is the only hormonal contraception where ovulation can still occur.

HOW DO I NAVIGATE THE TRANSITIONS BETWEEN PHASES?

Having four phases doesn't mean that you are reduced to only having four feelings, or that each phase will simply occur one after the other in an orderly fashion as though you'd flicked a nifty little switch. While you have four hormonal phases, the way you move into them is almost as important as being in the phase itself. This is useful to remember if you find yourself struggling with a particular phase. How was the phase before it? How well were you set up for this one?

YOUR POWERS ARE UNIQUE

So many factors make you who you are and determine how you respond to the bazillion things that happen in your life: your genes, your family, your living situation, your diet, how much time in nature you get, and your cycle. Like everything else about you, how you respond to your own hormones is unique. I'll be guiding you through how the four phases *might* make you feel, but everyone experiences them differently; some have challenges with different phases while others report few challenges at all. Having names for these four phases makes them real, and this is important when it comes to things you can't see, especially your emotions.

There are many ways to name your phases. In their book *Wild Power*, Alexandra Pope and Sjanie Hugo Wurlitzer connect the cycle (phases) to the seasons of the natural world. It was

Alexandra who originally saw this synchrony and began to speak of the inner seasons of the cycle.

In *The Optimized Woman*, Miranda Gray calls these phases Reflective, Dynamic, Expressive and Creative. If you are fond of considering your energy levels in terms of your f%ck budget, you might enjoy knowing this can also be applied to the cycle, too; zero f%cks, f%ck yes, f%cks for days and f%ck this.

You'll find you have an affinity with one or more of the phases, and they become like secret friends. 'Oh, hello, you,' you'll be saying in no time at all. 'I remember what I need to do now.' And even if you can't always give yourself what you need immediately, just knowing what it is that you need will provide deep relief. This is where the art of truly being a period queen comes through: in knowing your signs and what they're telling you. Week by week, month by month, you will learn more of your innate power. You will learn about what makes you tick, what makes you twitch and what makes your heart sing.

Look out, world! Period power coming through!

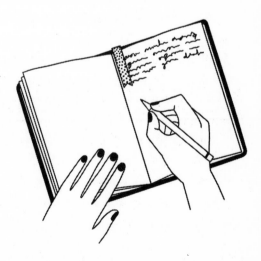

CHAPTER 4

DREAM

Imagine a queen who's made it down the mountain that was her last month to a lush, peaceful valley. The sun is setting behind her, and her legs feel like lead as she takes slow, deliberate steps towards the entrance of a cave. *Fiiiinally*, she thinks to herself, *I'm so fecking ready for this.* A warm fire crackles in the centre, and in the corner she spies a freshly made bed with a big, feathery duvet and chocolate on the pillow. She cries one happy tear and feels her shoulders soften — she's home. The sounds of the outside world fade away as she sinks into the bed and into the softest parts of herself. She begins to bleed. She knows she has powerful intuition now and that the best way to prepare for the month ahead is to listen to it. She knows how to dream.

Welcome to your bleed. No, really, welcome! Particularly if you are currently menstruating as you read this (quietly ensuring the survival of our species and bleeding away the life-giving nest within you). Welcome. You made it.

This is the very beginning of your cycle, and where you'll meet your first superpower: the power to dream. Maybe you arrived at this point a little bedraggled, but now you are here — back at the beginning of yourself. Know that Mother Nature wants nothing more than to hold you close, wrap you up in love and treat you with complete tenderness. Think of this Dream phase as the bedrock of your month because if you get this one right and bleed well, everything else will flow (quite literally).

What you are doing is no small thing.* To let go like this, the way we do almost every month, is not a chore to be rushed. Why would you rush when instead you could set yourself up for a good month and enjoy the beautiful benefits of this time?

That's right. This is the perfect time to enjoy ultimate self-care and press pause on life's non-essentials.

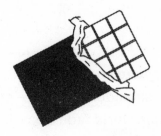

*And if you're doing it right now, hugs.

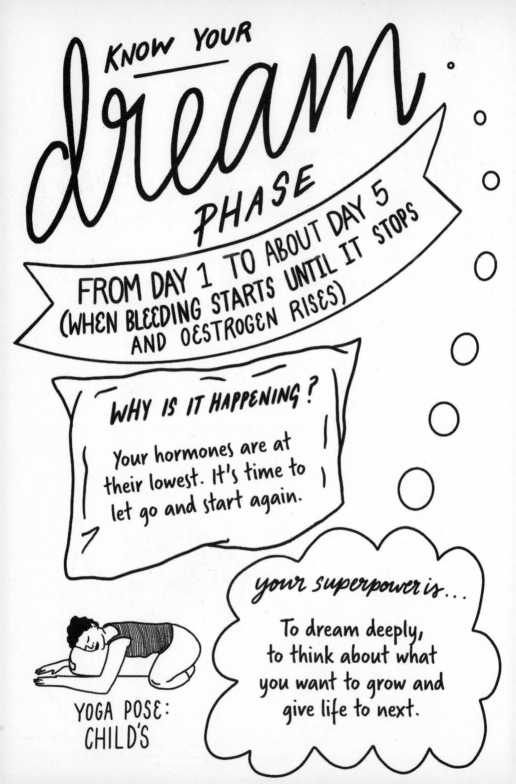

KNOW YOUR

dream

PHASE

FROM DAY 1 TO ABOUT DAY 5
(WHEN BLEEDING STARTS UNTIL IT STOPS
AND OESTROGEN RISES)

WHY IS IT HAPPENING?

Your hormones are at their lowest. It's time to let go and start again.

your superpower is...

To dream deeply, to think about what you want to grow and give life to next.

YOGA POSE: CHILD'S

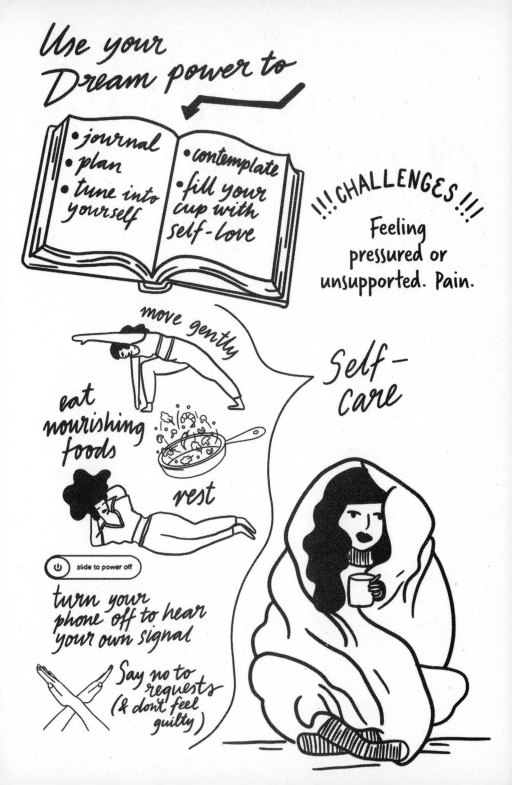

GET TO KNOW YOUR DREAM PHASE

There's a very precious power to be harnessed in your Dream phase, but to get even a glimpse of it, just a mere *whiff*, you need to let it come to you in its own sweet way. It's a quieter kind of power: the kind that can easily go unnoticed if it isn't made to feel welcome. Intuition doesn't waste itself on those who don't care for it. If you want it, you will need to be patient, but it is worth it.

The more you can be kind and love the bejeepers out of yourself while you are bleeding, the more you will begin to understand (and to maximise) the inherent loveliness of the Dream phase gifts. As well as the belief that you deserve this treatment, you also need time and space, which isn't always easy to come by. In fact, it can feel impossible to find at times. To futureproof yourself, preparation is key. Do some scaffolding and planning for this phase, and once you're in it you'll find there are lots of special ways to take care of your Dream self.

Hopefully, you'll savour this time. The cherry on the top is allowing your deep intuition to guide you. This is how you really crack the code of the menstrual power to Dream.

As your period comes to an end, you'll feel the dreaminess lift and the bubbling urge to Do. For now, be patient with your sweet self. Go as slowly and with as much self-love as you can muster. Next week will be different because when you are a cyclical creature, it always is.

SURRENDER TO DREAMING

When you stop fighting the 'big slow', you can accept it and, better still, you can actually enjoy it. I haven't always done it this well myself. Before I learned how to period, mine would come and I would groan and think, *Ergh, what a drag.* Now, I look back with compassion at my younger self who told her body that it was a drag, and I practise as much loveliness as I can to make up for it. When you do this, your period can actually be great — so great it might even take you by surprise.

Listen to this: after pitching *My Greatest Period Ever* to a room of theatre investors, a networking session followed. Everyone had name tags and business cards, and talked animatedly over biscuits and tea. A young woman made a beeline for me and said, 'I loved your pitch! And, um, do you want to know something really weird?'

I get this sort of question a lot and am always delighted by what people will share with me after all of four seconds. 'Of course!' I said.

She leaned in and whispered loudly, her eyes darting over my shoulders, presumably to monitor who might overhear: 'Look, I know this might sound strange, but I just finished my period, and it was . . .'

I nodded and waited while she searched for the right words until her expression landed on incredulous: ' . . . *so nice.* My whole period was really *nice!* I just relaxed and had a really good bleed and I wanted to tell everyone about it but I didn't know who to tell. I didn't know it could be like that.'

But now she does.

The beauty of having a lovely bleed is that once you know you can, you will expect to in the future. And so you should. It's not weird at all to have a nice bleed. Rather, it's weird that we would think it's weird. Of course you should have a lovely bleed and tell people if you feel like it. This is obviously a much better mindset than anticipating that your period or your body is going to be a drag. Nothing gets past your body — she's always listening.

HONOUR THE TRANSITION INTO DREAM

- ♥ Stock up on dark chocolate.
- ♥ Start drinking lovely herbal tea out of a favourite mug.
- ♥ Change your sheets.
- ♥ Have a long shower or a bath.
- ♥ Light a candle.

- 💜 Meditate.

- 💜 Turn your phone off, and imagine turning yourself to power-saving mode, too.

- 💜 Have a nap and/or give yourself ten minutes to stare out the window and watch the clouds with your feet up.

- 💜 Avoid tight waistbands and wear a mumu instead.

- 💜 Go 'under' with a duvet and some 'movie therapy'.

DREAM PHASE ESSENTIALS

- 💜 Hot water bottle, wheat pack or obliging pet

- 💜 Bleeding playlist to relax or meditate with

- 💜 Relaxing essential oils such as lavender, rose, chamomile and jasmine to rub onto your tummy/temples/wrists

- 💜 Warm dressing gown or some menstrual fashion that is floaty and comfortable

- 💜 Thick socks or Ugg boots

- 💜 Journal (to write in but also to read from)

- 💜 Eye mask

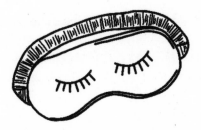

TRACKING YOUR DREAM PHASE

Given that you always know when you are bleeding, this phase should be the easiest to track. If knowing approximately when your period is due is all you keep track of for a while, that's okay — you're starting your understanding of your cycle at the best place. Use a journal or an app to note your Day 1 and pay attention to how many days you bleed for, and how you feel on each day. Your period might come on quite heavily or you could get more of a slow fade in, but the true beginning of your Dream phase is when you get actual blood (as opposed to any spotting for a day or two). If you do get spotting, definitely take that as a useful heads-up to start preparing for a good Dream phase.

Revisit the tracking tips on page 70.

UNLOCKING YOUR SUPERPOWER

Once your power is good and ready, it will arrive. The key to unlocking it lies in how you take care of yourself during this time (and in the lead up to it). Your needs on Day 1 will be different to your needs on Day 3, and your needs will be different to mine, so use the following suggestions for prioritising, setting boundaries and self-care as a guide. Enjoy exploring how you can create a regular practice out of making yourself feel precious.

SLOW DOWN

In the rush to make everyone accept that periods are a normal part of life, we got caught up in insisting that we can do everything we normally do during our periods — and that we must! Doing backflips in white pants, and so on. The truth is, you've just slain a proverbial dragon (during your premenstrual Take phase). You deserve a medal, or at the very least a chance to slow down.

As your bleed kicks in, you cross over into a hormonal vacuum, and this drop in hormones affects everything. No one else knows (unless you tell them, and please do) what you're doing on the inside. And therein lies the challenge: what with work, study, family, friends and life, there are so many reasons to push through. I'm not suggesting you need to spend a whole week on the couch meditating in a onesie (though that sounds like something we should all try once in our lives. No judgment here, you do you), but it's time to S L O W down. **The revolution will only be won with well-rested women.**

You can still 'do' life with a period; you just need to do it on your terms wherever possible. Just because you *can* force yourself to do something doesn't mean that you *have* to. The more you can slow down now, when your body really wants to, the more of everything you'll have in store for the month ahead. Instead of hitting your next phase on empty, you'll sail in ready to go, with a full cup of dreams and energy. So here's a hot tip: **you do not need to do it all right now, and you do not need to do it at 100 per cent.** Slow the heck down and *plan* for slowness in the same way you'd plan for an exciting adventure.

Start your day with a luxurious stretch in bed and yawn loudly to remind your body what moving luxuriously sounds like. Get up slowly and choose comfortable clothes. While you are having breakfast, brushing your teeth or looking for your keys, avoid behaving aerobically. Are you rushing? Do you need to? As you move through your day, take slower steps and deeper breaths. There is real joy in surrendering to that slowness and mental stillness that your body craves.

MAKE TIME

Sit down with your diary and draw some clouds around your period due date, perhaps with a day on either side. Keep these scheduled slow days as free as possible; with minimal pressure, you'll be able to care for yourself when the time comes.

If you know your period is due while you are on a holiday, don't despair because you can't prance around in a bikini or go rock climbing (because you can if you get enough rest). Rather, take the opportunity for a total dream queen experience. Pack a portable self-care kit with all the things you can think of to make you feel supported. Spend your days relaxing and dreaming, and see if this fills you with bliss.

Alternatively, if you've had the month from hell then you can be sure that your upcoming period is going to cost you more than usual in the self-care department. Start saving for this and build in extra buffers for time and space — see this as medicine you're stockpiling. Then, instead of dreading your period, you can look forward to it as a time to decompress, and you'll thank yourself later that you were able to.

MEDITATE

Relaxation, meditation, mindfulness — we know these things are all good for us, but we don't always feel like doing them because life gets busy. And exciting. But if we never got to slow down it wouldn't be as fun to go so fast, so thank goodness for the Dream phase. You are primed for meditating now, so if you've always wanted to start a practice, this is the time.

REST

Being busy is routinely rewarded over resting, but deep down your body knows the truth: even superwomen need rest. In fact, women are super *because* we rest. When you prioritise resting, you invest in your formidable future self. If you don't, the knock-on effects can last for weeks. Just like doing yoga or having a swim in the ocean, you will never regret getting quality rest. Even if you have a looming deadline and are prone to panicking, consider resting an investment that will help you get the most bang for your buck when you do sit down to get the job done.

So wherever possible, rest. At the very least, you should aim to get to bed slightly earlier and wake up slightly later this week because now you really do need more sleep and without it, everything will feel harder. If you can negotiate a pyjama day at home in lieu of going to work/uni/looking after kids or dealing with your life — do it! If you can't, there's always next month.

Use the tips on these pages to squeeze in whatever form of sweet, deep rest you can get. First things first, turn your phone to airplane mode or off. If you need to, tell whomever you share space with that you are having some time alone. Make yourself completely comfortable in the following fashion (or in whichever fashion you deem conducive to getting the deepest rest).

💜 Take a hot shower or a bath.

💜 If you feel any body aches that might stop you from being able to relax, start with a few stretches.

💜 Have a warm, milky drink (milk contains tryptophan, an amino acid that helps to induce sleep).

💜 Get yourself a hot water bottle if you need one.

💜 Set a timer before shutting your eyes. This will help you to relax as you won't be worried about sleeping for too long. If you don't actually sleep, rest assured that what you are doing is almost as good and still excellent preparation for whatever you need to do next.

💜 Imagine someone gently placing a magnificent dressing gown — heavy and soft, velvet, lined with smooth silk — around your shoulders.

💜 Put drops of lavender oil on the pillow to soothe your senses.

💜 Snuggle up in bed and lie on your back under a weighted blanket or heavy blankets to make you feel held.

💜 Put a pillow under your knees to take the pressure off your lower back if you have any pain there.

💜 Cover your eyes with an eye mask or a soft cotton T-shirt so that no light gets in. Soften your face.

💜 Slow down your breathing and try to enjoy stretching out the space between breathing out and breathing in again.

💜 Scan your body from head to toe. Notice if you are 'holding on' to any tension. Is it in your forearms, or your hands? Are you literally still holding on? Is it in your hips? Are you bracing yourself for an imaginary fall?

💜 Let your arms and legs fall apart gently, and roll your limbs out back and forth a few times. Take a deep breath and hold them as far out as they'll comfortably go. Imagine everything turning outwards, your hips and shoulders opening, and then exhale slowly as your limbs melt back to their most comfortable position.

💜 If you come across any parts of your lovely self that are tight or achy, breathe into them. Spend several breaths sending love and softness to anywhere that needs it, and feel your body go deeper and deeper into rest.

💜 Imagine a hundred tiny hands tenderly squeezing away any little aches and pains.

💜 Remind yourself that you are safe. You are warm in your bed, and all you need to do now is allow this replenishing rest.

💜 When it's time to get up, feel your fingers touching each other, stretch your body out like a cat and then roll onto your right side before sitting, giving your heart one last moment to enjoy less pressure while it rests above your other organs.

Feel how every cell in your body has been given a chance to recalibrate. Imagine a layer of calm around you as you move through your day and then revisit this space anytime you want with a deep breath.

NURTURE YOURSELF

To really use this Dream time wisely, and to lean in and to surrender to it, one does not simply just *rest*. My friends, this is the time to nurture yourself. If only on your heaviest day, it is important to treat yourself preciously while your body is doing such important work. Nurture yourself like your life depends on it because the quality of your month ahead certainly does.

Normally, bleeding (from a non-vaginal area) elicits helpful behaviour from others such as the offering of assistance, a bandaid or a cup of tea. You would think that after many, many periods, I would be used to it by now, but I still occasionally experience a small shock at the sight of my own bright blood and feel that some sort of assistance would be greatly appreciated. Where is my cup of tea?

I wish for a future where every menstruator has someone to make them tea, someone to take a load off (or put a load on), to cook them dinner and run them a bath. If this kind of support is available to you, enjoy it but see it as icing on a cake that you still have to make yourself.

Twelve times a year we are given this opportunity for true self-love, so be generous with yourself, whether that means dining in the bath on precooked lasagne (for breakfast, lunch and/

or dinner), rubbing scented oil into your damp skin or watching a sunset and drinking it in. Make and take every chance for tenderness, and if support isn't forthcoming, rub your own feet. Stroke your own forehead, like you would a child.

If you catch yourself feeling like you aren't a big deal and thinking that you should have a coffee and a painkiller and soldier on, please remind yourself that you are so deserving of this tenderness. If you get your period just before a long drive home after a wedding down south, opt for the scenic route even if it takes a bit longer. If you happen to drive through a forest of the biggest, most majestic trees in your state, get out and sit underneath one knowing that you are safe and precious and a part of life's mystery and plan. Breathe.

And if, after this journey, you have another one on a red-eye flight that lands at 5 am on the day of your opening night of a two-week run of shows, consider your options for nurturing very, very carefully. There's only so much pressure that yoga and lavender oil can ameliorate. When this exact recipe for disaster became a reality for me, I did something I'd never done before: I upgraded our flights. Those precious hours of sleep, in a seat that turned into a bed, under a duvet, with a pillow, socks and an eye mask, were some of the best and most needed in my life. If you are able, treat yourself at such critical junctures. If not then, when?

SURVIVING OUT IN THE WORLD

Inevitably, at some point during our Dream phase we will need to be out in the real world, interacting with real people and doing real things. You can still do this and honour where you're at with a repertoire of survival strategies:

💜 Take a hot water bottle with you (with a cover so the heat will last for hours). When I rehearse with my lovely band on Days 1–3, I'll sit instead of standing, with a hot water bottle tucked into my trackpants. When I ask if we can play half as loud, no one ever minds — they often like this break, too.

💜 Use headphones and some classical music when you need to focus in a busy co-working space.

💜 Where possible, avoid protracted conversations (you are on emotional skeleton staff; hide if necessary).

💜 In a meeting, take the comfiest chair available and do not offer to take the minutes.

💜 If there is a conflict to be resolved, allow space for others to get into the fray and take the path of least resistance.

💜 Smile serenely (for your own benefit) and take your time to respond when people ask you questions. Don't let anyone rush you. You are on Dream time and your body will thank you for this simple practice.

💜 When a nice thing is offered, be it a favour, cake (the biggest piece obviously has your name on it), tea or to go first in a line, accept it graciously.

♥ Better still, ask for help. This is your time to do the asking. If instead someone asks you for help that is non-essential to his or her immediate survival, consider yourself temporarily unavailable. You'll have time to give soon enough.

♥ When you get home, a nap and/or bath can cure almost anything, or at the very least take the hard edges off. You did it — a day in the world while bleeding. Now collapse onto a soft surface for more dreaming.

DO SOME YOGA

Moving and stretching your body helps you to let go of whatever you need to so you can connect more fully with yourself and allow your dreams to bubble to the surface. Try different classes until you find a style of yoga you connect with. There are so many variations, you can even look online and practise at home.

Yin is a peaceful, slow, supported style of yoga that uses lots of props to make you comfortable. It often includes singing bowls and sound baths (very menstrual). Then there's also yoga nidra, which translates to 'sleep yoga'. It's like medicine for your body and will make you feel loved in your bones.

Wherever you are, you can always take a big yoga breath. Breathe deeply from your womb up into your chest. Feel your rib cage expand as the sides of your lungs fill, then *riiight* up . . . up, up, up into the top of your chest. Hold it for just a few seconds and feel your collarbones expand before emptying your lungs from the very top all the way back down into your womb. A big beautiful breath is always available to you.

LISTEN TO YOUR DREAMS

In the day: Find a few little windows to daydream. If you feel the need to lie on the grass with the sun on your back, then that is exactly what you should do — even if only for ten minutes. With bare feet in the grass, or up against a tree, enjoy feeling more grounded and connected to the Earth, where millions and millions of women have been menstruating and communing with themselves for thousands of years, just like you are now. If you can be in nature, you'll be more inclined to notice little signs, such as a breath of wind or a bird flying by or an interestingly shaped cloud. Like omens, these signs remind you to remember your dreams.

In the night: Notice your sleeping dreams as well. While you are sleeping, everything else melts away and the cream rises to the top. The best way to remember dreams is to decide as you are falling asleep that you really want to. Reassure your body that you are *listening*. Write them down as soon as you wake up, and don't worry if they don't immediately make sense. During the day the messages in the dream will keep working on you, and you will start to piece together some meaning. Sometimes, the meanings are pretty obvious.

Day 1 Dream Journal

I dreamed I was climbing up a cliff with one hand and dragging a suitcase with the other, overlooking a wild ocean on a bright sunny day with big, fluffy clouds. Finally, I got up to the top and was just about to use the last of my energy to haul up the suitcase when I realised I didn't want the damn thing anymore, and I hurled it into the sea.

SUSTAINABLE PERIODS

While we're on the topic of being in the world while bleeding, we should talk about how best (for you and the planet) to catch the blood in question. Thankfully, re-usable period products are becoming more and more available and accepted the world over, and their benefits are significant. Not only are they so much better for the environment, your body and your wallet, you also avoid the association between yourself and your lovely body and the production of rubbish, to be hidden and disposed of. You can buy period pants and re-usable pads made of soft, comfortable material to be worn again and again. You can even make simple ones out of folded flannelette cotton squares.

Granted, washing them yourself is a little more effort than wrapping up a tampon or a pad to go in the bin. When I first started using and washing re-usable pads and period pants, I was very aware of how it felt to have my hands in the bloody water that had come from my body. But now I see the vivid red as symbolic of my power in all of its rich glory. It makes me feel reverent and grateful; so does knowing how much unnecessary waste I'm avoiding. Every year, in Australia alone, 300 million tampons and 500 million pads go into landfill, where each one will take up to 800 years to break down. Every conventional pad and tampon ever bought and used is yet to break down. If you choose cotton biodegradable tampons, they will take around six months to decompose.

If I'm travelling, the solution is a cup. Menstrual cups, made of silicone and inserted in much the same way as a tampon, are becoming more popular, but, like tampons, using them can take some getting used to. I bought one with good intentions as soon as I discovered they existed, but the thing sat in my bathroom cupboard for almost two years. I pulled it out every now and again and struggled with getting it to feel right until, *finally,* I got the hang of it. Now I absolutely love it and use it exclusively while I'm away from home (sometimes with a liner on a heavy day).

Menstrual cups don't soak up your vaginal fluids like tampons do, so they don't dry you out on a light day, which causes some people considerable discomfort. You can leave them in (depending on your flow) for up to 8 hours or overnight if you want to. Cleaning them is quick and easy. If, like me, you initially find the idea of inserting and removing a cup daunting, I recommend trying one — if only to better become acquainted with your own anatomy. Once you've used it a few times, you'll start to know your shape and space.

Managing blood flow from an intimate area of your body can feel like a bother, but consider experimenting with re-usables and making this process into its own self-care ritual. I sing while I wash out my pads now.

USE YOUR DREAM PHASE POWER

The reward for all of this self-care is the power to dream — to daydream, to night dream and to *deep* dream. This is a time to tune in to your deepest self, to your intuition and your biggest dreams. You can use what you discover in powerful ways. Here are some suggestions.

TO GUIDE YOUR LIFE

As you walk the line between an old month and a brand shiny new one, your intuition is at its strongest, so make sure you listen to it and use it to guide your new month. What do you want to grow and give life to next? Is there something you want to focus on? How do you want this next month to look?

While you're at it, what do you want your whole life to look like? Planning for how you want to feel as you look back over your life is a nice way to guide yourself. Imagine what inspiration and advice your ninety-year-old self might have for you. She would undoubtedly tell you not to worry what other people think and to chase down your best dreams.

TO BIRTH NEW IDEAS

Your blood arriving is the signal that your time to dream has begun, so get ready for the insights because you are never more connected to the source (*sauce, ha*) than now. While you are bleeding and being slow and gentle on the outside, all of your new ideas are bubbling away and percolating on the inside. Along with your developing eggs, your precious idea babies will be ready to emerge fully formed once your Dream phase is over and they've been bathed in stillness.

Dream deeply and consider that you are investing in fabulous ideas for the month ahead. When you get a fabulous idea, write it down to make it real. These dreams are the beginnings of your stories and your next adventures. Catch them gently on the page. If something feels like a big YES to you right now, your body, mind and soul really mean it. So don't mess around.

Obviously with great dreams come great responsibility, and yes, you will need to work for them in order to make them come alive. But you don't need to run just yet. You'll do that in the following two phases. For now, you're purpose-built to collect dreams and ideas. Your job is to sift through them — to figure out which ones to hold close and to find the heroes worth fighting for. This is NOT the time to put a lid on yourself or your imagination.

TO REVISIT OLD IDEAS

Big, fabulous *old* ideas need some quiet time for rumination every month, too. Some projects or quandaries will be with you for many cycles, bubbling away on the backburner. During the Dream phase, take the lid off them and see how they're coming along. Add a pinch of this and that, and give them a stir. Maybe they need another cycle; good things take time. If you feel like you're going around in circles with something, you are! You're meant to. That's the beauty of having a cycle and four phases to help you move through your life.

Journalling about your dreams and deep feelings can serve as your anchor throughout the month. Coming back to these writings and remembering what spoke to you in your Dream phase will help you to feel grounded and connected to your deepest self. This is a good practice to follow as you finish bleeding and prepare to move more into the world again (before Do).

TO DO AN EMOTIONAL CHECK-IN

Our cycle asks us to stop before we start again. Without this contemplative time we'd run to keep up, push to get through and end up missing the precious signposts of the Dream phase. Then, before you know it, it's time to Do again (at pre-ovulation) and you are swept back to the surface with new demands, opportunities and temptations without having had time to digest the ones still on your plate from last month. There is nothing as sad as a half-baked dream left to wither when you really still want it. Do you still want it? It's never too late.

Nature has built in this pause for a reason, and without it we feel overloaded. Now that you know this, you can use this time for what it is truly meant for. As you sink into the sanctity of your period and allow your feelings, whatever shape they take, to just be, you tune in to the most ancient wisdom of all. After a few days of this emotional spaciousness, your deepest feelings are no longer glimmers that you can't quite place. They have a weight now; they are ready to be seen and measured. Held in the palm of your hand.

For a few months, I pondered whether to perform at Perth Fringe Festival again. With each period, I explored this question from a different angle: should I do my show in its current form or a different version? Should I write a whole new show? Should I not do it at all? It took almost four months to come to the right conclusion. I *would* write a new show, but not for another year. This time I would work with a director. It was well worth the wait.

TO LET GO

It takes time to clear your plate (physically, as well as emotionally). Sitting quietly, lying in a bath or under a tree, is where we do this work.

Once you've had a good look at everything, decide what you want to keep and what you're ready to let go of. When your womb is soft and letting go of that lovely nest, your mind and your heart can follow suit if you let them. I like to call this your 'biological verge pick-up' because along with your endometrial lining, you can also let go of anything else you don't need mentally or emotionally. Why would you want to drag a whole suitcase of junk you don't need anymore into a brand new month? Chuck it. Biff it over the cliff. Whatever it is, give voice to it and say out loud what it is that you want to release, or write it down and then burn the paper, or sing in the shower and wash it down the drain.

This is also the time to decide *not* to let something go because it definitely needs tending to. One of the best ways to work out what to throw on the pile and what to hold on to or explore further is to use your Dream phase as a filter.

TO RUN TRUTH BOMBS THROUGH YOUR DREAM FILTER

Truth bombs are commonly uncovered during the Take (pre-menstrual) phase. Ominous, fizzing and threatening to erupt in your face, these need to be handled carefully. Managing them is a two-part process. Firstly, to relieve your premenstrual self of having to work it all out in the moment, write the truth bomb down. It's still there, but it's temporarily disarmed.

Current pop culture would have us believe that it's quite normal to feel 'crazy' and 'psycho' before we get our period, and then go 'back to normal' once it arrives. But consider another way of looking at these strong emotions: perhaps you've been putting up with some crap all month long and your body, mind and soul have finally reached their maximum crap capacity. Perhaps this 'craziness' is a protective mechanism so you'll have less crap to deal with while you are actually bleeding.

And now that you are bleeding, it's time for the second part of the process: considering and addressing the truth bomb with fresh eyes and an emptying womb. This is a good activity for Day 3 or 4. This same process can also be applied to anything big that you aren't sure how to move forward with.

Here's how it's done:

1. First, look back over any truth bombs you recorded when you were premenstrual (more on this in Chapter 7, Take) and check the weight of them now. If something bothered you enough for you to write it down and it still bothers you now, while you are letting go, then this unsatisfactory situation or truth bomb is as bad/almost as bad/potentially worse than you suspected. *Especially* if the same gripe has been popping up over a few cycles, it is not 'just your hormones'. It is definitely a real thing.

2. So, it's real. What to do? Now that you've acknowledged that this issue requires addressing, the best way forward is to bleed on it. How would you like this situation to look or feel instead? Sit with it and imagine how you might reshape it. Using some of the aforementioned resting tips, make yourself comfortable and allow your mind to become clear.

   While you can do this any time, it's easiest when you have your period — when you are closest to your heart. Let all the possible solutions come and go and wash over you. Pay attention when one lands on the right spot and gives you a feeling of relief, like a little key finding the right lock. When you say, 'Ah ha', believe yourself; your gut's reaction is your womb wisdom. Those are golden nuggets.

3. Don't worry if a solution doesn't come straight away. Maybe you need to talk about it with someone you can trust to get some ideas, maybe you just need to talk out loud and hear the sound of your own voice. I sometimes do this on a voice memo while on long drives, and as I'm speaking, I hear the solution tumble out. Notice and be open and receptive to signs.

4. Ideas and solutions will come eventually, and they don't need to be perfect. You just need to feel that you are going to do *something* to address this thing that is clearly an issue. And maybe you'll need to address it a few times before you conquer it.

5. Once you have an idea for a solution, should you rush out and execute it? Well, you could. Or you could schedule it for a few days' time, once you're in your Do phase. You'll feel more energetic then and have the confidence to take things on. That said, if the situation requires maximum sensitivity and delicate handling, consider scheduling it for the Give phase, see Chapter 6 (that's the best time to tackle difficult conversations).

6. Dealing with difficult situations is really hard (for everyone). Now you've given it your best shot. Well done. Every time you do this, your intuition grows stronger. Keep at it, sister.

TO FORGE DEEP CONNECTIONS

With all this self-care and dreaming, you might find yourself feeling exceptionally connected — to yourself, to your loved ones, to the cosmos, to everything. We are made to come together at this time with other women so we can connect deeply and learn from (and of) each other. Spending time with people you don't have to try with, whether that's in a circle or on the phone, is where contemplation happens, too. We mirror each other. I partially credit my current emotional intelligence to all those times when I'd stay home at the beginning of my period and spend the day drinking cups of tea with Mum and watching *Oprah*. Little did I know how much I was learning in our little circle. Me, mum and Oprah.

If you feel a bittersweet ache in your chest during this phase and the only thing for it is to cry–sing along to sad girl music in the dark, then open your curtains and see if the moon will join you. If you feel sad, feel sad! It will pass eventually and you don't need to push through it, just like you don't need to push through your period. So feel it, go there. Light a candle and sink into it (the feeling, not the candle). Don't brace against it. Let it wash over you, and enjoy all of the colours of your emotional rainbow. The world will happen around you and all over you. Let it. Stay soft; you're stronger like this.

You might like to write or express yourself with art, music or dance, which is also good for any pain. Sometimes I write songs when I'm feeling like this, and it feels good to use my body to amplify what I'm feeling. Western culture doesn't encourage us to engage with sadness, but the more you honour these feelings the less you need to fear them. If it's in there, let it out.

Sometimes during this phase I watch Richard moving around our kitchen in his dressing gown — cleaning it up or making tea for me while I lie on the couch — and I feel so deeply appreciative of being held and cared for, and so full of love for him. I tell him how much I appreciate all that he does for me and I feel so grateful to be held by my body, and to be sharing it with someone special. If you are well supported, this can be an exquisite time to connect and be tender with a partner. Blissful even.

Other times, perhaps when *I'm* moving around the kitchen and wishing I could sit down under the shower instead, I feel less grateful. If you don't feel supported during this time, you can feel unseen and broken-hearted. But don't despair. Remember that your most important relationship is with yourself, so give to yourself, and reflect on whether there is truth in your feelings of abandonment. This is your most vulnerable time, and your partner/family members need to learn this. Let them know where you are in your cycle and what that means; help them understand. If they care about you, they will. Ask for help, be specific about what you need and you can return the favour during your Give phase. It isn't always easy to be vulnerable and to receive. Now is your chance.

PLAY TO YOUR STRENGTHS AT WORK

The great thing about your body slowing down is that your brain gets a rest, too. You have less of a 'monkey mind' and more of an 'elephant mind' — wise and observant (maybe also bloated). But can you still be productive when you are trying to slow down to match the pace of your menstrual cycle? How do you deal with stressful situations at work when just wearing pants is a struggle? The answer is scaffold, scaffold (nap) and scaffold.

You can still do what you need to do in this phase, but not without self-care and definitely not if you spend your energy budget helping other people with their jobs or processing emotional palavers from the weekend. Put one foot in front of the other, and remember that done is better than perfect. If you're about to leave and your boss asks, 'Is there anyone who can stay back?' keep your head down and make a beeline for that door. In the meantime, believe it or not, there's a lot to be gained from working in the Dream phase.

TACKLING PROJECTS

Assuming you are working to a deadline but have a bit of time up your sleeve, start with some constructive dreaming. This is the groundwork that prepares the soil before you can grow something fabulous. Mull over research material, watch videos or listen to podcasts to help you understand more about the topic at hand and the direction you might take. Make notes that you can come back to when you are ready to rumble. You'll feel less pressured and more in sync with yourself if you have time to gather your thoughts and massage them into shape. Trust that your intuition will allow you to join the dots into the big picture.

When you can, batch mentally onerous tasks that require critical thinking in a day or two. If they have to be done in this phase, allow more time than you normally would for them. Above all, remind yourself that you are more than enough, even at 64 per cent capacity.

HAVING TO DO SOMETHING HARD WHEN YOU'RE BLOODY WELL BLEEDING

What if you do need to be on top of your game mid-bleed? Good news: you can do whatever you want, whenever you want as long as you prepare. If you leave a presentation or an assignment to the last minute and that last minute just happens to coincide with you getting your period, it can really suck. Feeling pressured is the last thing you need, so be realistic about what you can achieve and how. Don't expect to be able to wing things as easily as you normally might because you are not in top slaying mode (although it might feel like your womb is).

However, in saying that, if you've been able to scaffold suffi-ciently, you might surprise yourself. And, for a limited time, you may be able to actually slay quite well or even better than usual on account of the extra rest you've been getting. But if you were too busy or sick to scaffold and now you're deep in the Dream phase and expected to deliver or else, try this: firstly, take a deep breath. Oxygenating yourself is always a good idea, particularly when you are feeling overwhelmed or anxious.

Remind yourself that it's going to be okay. Consider asking for help from someone not in the same hormonal condition (possibly in their Give phase). At least your care factor acts as immunity to things that might otherwise annoy you, such as someone asking a question that makes a meeting go for an extra 20 minutes or Darren's friendly reminder emails. Drop your shoulders as well as any expectations that you must give 100 per cent of yourself 100 per cent of the time. Even people without periods don't do that. Get enough sleep and breakfast, pack your portable self-care unit and carry yourself (in stretchy pants) with the 'confidence of a mediocre white dude', as writer Sarah Hagi so brilliantly tweeted in 2015. Don't forget, anything he can do, you can do bleeding. You just might need a nap after, and maybe a wine . . . in the bath. Give your arm a little stroke and now do the blinking thing as best as you can.

On my first day of bleeding I prefer to be at home alone, but often my period arrives right before I go on stage. I've learned not to be afraid of this; while I might take a bit longer to warm up, being at my most vulnerable is a beautiful gift to share. This happened to a friend of mine, an incredible soul singer named Odette Mercy, during a concert with a symphony orchestra.

At rehearsal before opening night, she seemed a little tired and wasn't belting out her songs like she normally does. 'Day 1', she said to me, with a knowing nod. The next night, I watched from the wings while she sang Adele's 'Someone Like You' with the crowd in the palm of her hand. By the final chorus, they were singing along and then, all of a sudden, Odette stopped. Completely overcome with emotion, she blanked on the lyrics. It happens occasionally, and performers usually recover quickly before anyone notices. Not this time. As the audience sang their hearts out to her *'I wish nothing but the best for youuuuu, tooooo!'* her heart overflowed, along with her tears. It was the sweetest moment of the night. Whether it's with 1000 people or just one, it can be very special when you feel safe enough to let others see your softness.

What a thing to be a human woman gifted with this full emotional spectrum. How fortunate for your workplace that they can benefit from this, from your tenderness. When you go to work, whatever your job is, never forget that you are a human being, not just a human doing. As always, be where you are.

Odette and I have a fabulous mutual friend, Lucy Hopkins (an activist/priestess/clown/witch/deity). Her favourite thing to say is, 'Why not?'. But my favourite thing she ever said was about the Dream phase: 'Be not afraid of your great depth, for therein is your greatest power.'

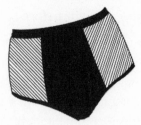

CHALLENGES IN THE DREAM PHASE

Humans have evolved in part due to our altruistic nature; being kind to each other has helped us survive. There are times to be kind to others and times to be kinder to yourself, but living with the expectation of kindness in a fast-paced society that rewards constant productivity means it can be difficult to make the distinction. There are challenges to navigate in this phase if we want to avoid unnecessary emotional and physical suffering.

SAYING NO AND SETTING BOUNDARIES

We prefer to please people than to cause disappointment, but saying yes without actually thinking about what is right for us can get us into hot water.

Make no mistake, you *can* do the things that are really important to you right now, but you can only do them well if you get the rest that you need and deserve. Putting something off because you have your period doesn't mean you are procrastinating, it means you are prioritising. By doing this, you're conserving your energy and you'll usually find that you have just enough in the tank to get done what is truly important to you.

If you are worried about letting people down, try letting them in on your deepest need or desire so they know what you're saying yes to instead. Explain that you have a limited energy budget right now. If it's someone you love, give them a choice: would you rather I visited your grandmother with you or picked up plants for the vegie patch? What friend or good-hearted person would begrudge you for this? Setting boundaries is a necessary skill in order to live the life that *you* actually want to live. You can't possibly say yes to everything, and if people are disappointed it really isn't up to you to fix that for them. They choose how to feel, not you.

On the other hand, saying no to something you really would like to do at any other time is much harder. If an opportunity presents itself and you are mid heavy bleed but feeling in two minds, remember, if you *really* want to do it so much that you can justify slotting it into your essential pile, that's fine. But it means something *else* will get bumped. You can do it all, but you can't do it all right now.

If it's hard to know what you want, say you'll think about it. This is a key phrase in the lexicon of a queen who knows how to period. Very powerful words they are, because they *buy you time* — time to consider whether this request from the outside world fits into the essential or the non-essential pile. If something seems like an unmissable idea, ask yourself, *Do I have FOMO? What will this cost? Does it have to be now? Do I feel pressured?*

Next week you'll be firing on all cylinders (if you commit to getting enough rest now), so you can confidently book a few things in, knowing that you'll have more energy then. Saying no and setting boundaries can be hard, but we absolutely have to do it. If you don't, you are effectively saying no to yourself instead. So start saying it and, while you're at it, don't apologise.

THE GUILTS

Feeling guilty is the number one enemy of the Dream phase; it's often what makes us say yes when we want to say no. And the worst thing about guilt? It's not even productive. It gets in the way of what we *really* need to do, *as well as* what we feel we 'should' be doing.

In a society that doesn't place enough value on resting, we have to actively unlearn this tendency towards guilt and rewire ourselves for rest. If you notice yourself feeling guilty for going slower or doing less, remind yourself that it's natural. Think about the seasons. Does a farmer feel guilty for slowing everything down in winter? Does a fruit tree for that matter? Imagine how depleted the soil would get if it was expected to be constantly productive. How poor the fruit. Actually, you don't even need to imagine; you can see for yourself the damage that's done when nature isn't permitted to rest and recover. A fruit tree doesn't feel guilty. It just does what it needs to do at the natural time to do it. So should you.

What can really help is paying attention to the way you talk to yourself. Every time you catch yourself thinking, *Oh, I should be doing this/that/some other thing,* ask yourself where this is coming from. Are you worried about what someone else thinks? Are you mistaking genuine self-care for laziness? Are you comparing yourself to others? Do you feel that you need to be doing things all of the time to be valuable?

Meet Ava. She's in Year 9, and she told me that the worst thing about having her period was feeling guilty every time she came home from school feeling completely zonked. She'd lie on the couch and do nothing until dinnertime, but instead of enjoying the rest she needed after a long day, she'd punish herself by thinking of all the things she *should* be doing.

Then at school the next morning, Ava would listen aghast as her friends chatted about their impressive achievements from the night before — replicating *MasterChef* meals or doing extension homework. She'd paste a smile on but inwardly feel even guiltier than she had the night before. *Ergh. I am the worst* she'd think to herself. Ava told me (with a glint in her eye) that now she thinks about resting in a completely different way: 'I just tell myself over and over that I deserve to rest. I tell myself that I don't need to feel guilty and then, eventually, I actually don't. Now when I have my period and I'm tired, I rest. Instead of feeling guilty, I *LOVE* it.'

Ava has rewritten her resting script, and so can you. If you didn't do a lot today other than period, then well done. The planet thanks you.

A PERIOD THAT'S GONE AWOL

This is all well and good if you are, in fact, bleeding. But what if you aren't? Regular menstruation and ovulation are signs that your body is in good health, so if you aren't cycling well there might be something else that needs investigating. Get to the bottom of what's going on with you, and see a good doctor — one who listens.

Although it's common to have wildly irregular periods because we commonly live in ways that don't support our cycles, it isn't normal. So if you are fed up because your cycle is irregular, it's worth learning more about how you can support your hormonal health. To that end, *Period Repair Manual* is a good place to start.

Remember that taking the pill to 'make your period regular' is a myth. It only works to mask any underlying factors, so if there is an actual problem you won't know what it is. The pill (and almost all other hormonal contraceptives) works by preventing ovulation. Without ovulation you don't have your own hormones or a true period at all, but rather a 'withdrawal bleed'. While you take the inactive sugar pills, your endometrium breaks down in response to the lack of synthetic hormones that maintain the lining in the absence of your own hormones.

Of course, you are still bloody well bleeding though, and if you are on the pill (or any hormonal contraception for that matter), you should 100 per cent employ the advice in this chapter and the self-care techniques. Pay attention to your feelings for any threads of meaning, for this is when you are most likely to feel and sense them as it's the only time that you don't take any synthetic hormones. Bleed away and read on.

If your period just decides from time to time to come late or not at all, THE most common culprit is stress. Think about it: the biological function of our cycle is to ensure the survival of the human species. From an evolutionary perspective, it made sense for stress to temporarily halt a woman's cycle: times of stress (caused by things such as invasions, war, food shortages or sabre-tooth tiger attacks) weren't the best times to be pregnant or have a baby. These days, our problems might not be quite so life and death, but the result of stress is the same: your body gets the message and your cycle goes on strike until things calm down. If you are too stressed, think about what's happening to your metaphorical babies (your big dreams and goals): they can't get born either because your body is in survival mode. In a nutshell, stress causes the production of cortisol, which interferes with ovulation.

Your cycle also relies on you ingesting sufficient carbohydrates and fats so it can afford to menstruate and possibly conceive and then breastfeed. Another very common reason for AWOL periods is that many people just don't eat enough, causing the body to also feel stress. Lastly, if you were on the pill and now you aren't, your period can take its sweet time to return and the wait can be very distressing. Whatever the reason for your periodic period, your body is trying to tell you something. Try not to feel frustrated. Instead, lather it with support. Even if you aren't bleeding, give yourself a Dream phase now more than ever.

MANAGING PAIN

By listening to your body and indulging in all that guilt-free slowness and self-love, you might find that garden-variety period pains are greatly eased or even eradicated altogether. It shouldn't come as a surprise that when we take the pressure off ourselves, we literally take the pressure off! We feel better. Your period can even be nice. But even if you do all the right things, your period can still hurt and pain can get in the way of you enjoying your slow week.

During your period (especially the first few days) you might feel quite tender. The main reason for this is inflammatory proteins called prostaglandins, which are made by the endometrial cells (womb lining) just before your period. Once your period starts, prostaglandins are released to stimulate the muscular layers of your womb to contract. This is very useful for helping your period to happen efficiently, but some of these prostaglandins can get into the nearby bloodstream in your abdominal area, causing you to experience the following not-so-nice things:

- Physical sensitivity: feeling tender and achy, low tolerance to pain. Don't subject yourself to any form of waxing now.

- A mild heaviness in your thighs and lower back, and/or belly bloating.

- A more intense, deep, brewing ache.

- Abdominal cramps as the layers of muscle that make up your womb twist and turn and squeeze to shed its innermost layer. These can range from minor cramps to 100 per cent what-the-hell-is-going-on cramps.

- Headaches and/or nausea.

- Diarrhoea. (Really? Yep.) It's as though your body knows it's about to get very busy letting go of your womb lining so before that begins in earnest it wants to get everything else off the table as well.

GET HELP FOR ABNORMAL PAIN

Pain can really cramp your style. Some people experience pain so badly that they start taking painkillers *before* their period even starts, just to prepare for its onset. Please don't feel you have to endure pain that gets in the way of you enjoying your life.

If you are suffering, you deserve answers and solutions. Although most doctors are benevolent people sufficiently educated in the menstrual cycle basics, not all are well versed in the nuances and subtleties of the menstrual experience. So if you speak to a doctor who isn't very helpful, they're not a good fit for you. Try another and don't stop looking until you find one who is helpful.

By tracking your cycle, you'll have collected valuable data on your body that will be useful for when you do find one. Unbearable pain and very heavy periods might be common, but that doesn't mean you should suffer in silence. There might be something else going on that needs medical attention.

If your pain is more of the normal variety, then here are a few other strategies to cope with it.

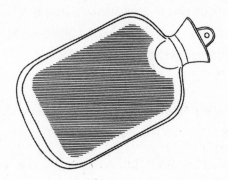

SEE THE PAIN AS A MESSAGE

Pain is common, but not normal. What is it telling you? What is your 'normal'? What does your body need? When you see any pain through the lens of self-care, it means you are more able to soften into it and see it as a request from your body. Instead of a warning, think about your pain as a message. Stay as soft as you can.

NUTRITION

Many traditional Chinese medicine practitioners agree it's quite weird how Western women believe that periods are meant to be painful. Dr Lara Briden blames dairy for the way our bodies respond with pain during our periods. If you suffer from painful periods, try eliminating dairy and noticing the results. In addition, taking zinc and magnesium supplements can help. Speak to a practitioner for more advice.

HOT WATER BOTTLES/HOT WHEAT BAGS

Whoever invented the hot water bottle surely has a special place in heaven. The combination of pressure and heat can work absolute wonders to alleviate pain. Any kind of heat will do, whether that's a wheat bag or standing against the oven in the kitchen. The other day I jumped on my bike and rediscovered the extra menstrual pleasure of a sun-warmed seat. Make a big mug of something delicious and rest it against your belly.

MEDITATE, MASTURBATE, MEDICATE

When all else fails, the phrase 'meditate, masturbate, medicate' comes to mind. While I'm not against the use of painkillers, this phrase, coined by Luna Matatas, a sex and pleasure educator in Toronto, Canada, is a good reminder that it also makes sense to use the natural options you have available to you.

Soften to the pain with meditation. When we physically brace ourselves, anticipating impact, we feel pain much more acutely. Quite simply, stress and tension make period pain worse. As I've mentioned, breathing is one of the most effective pain-management strategies, and so is meditation. Try listening to some relaxing music for meditation while you breathe into your belly and soften yourself — let go from every angle. Hopefully your body will get the message that it's being supported and can quit with the pain message being quite so intense.

As well as meditation, which lowers cortisol, touching your-self to the point of orgasm releases a bunch of good hormones. Orgasms are proven to bring relief from period pain. If you have endometriosis (which we'll discuss in a moment) then an actual orgasm when you are suffering can be too intense. But don't be deterred. Eloise, who'll you'll meet in the next chapter, described how finding her 'magic pain button' (clitoris) and gently rubbing it helped her to manage her pain. Be tender with yourself.

And then we medicate. Anti-inflammatories help slow down the production of the prostaglandins, which are what cause the contractions.* This will help in the short term, but in the long term consider taking magnesium and zinc as prophylactics, as they both also work to reduce inflammation.

*In Period Repair Manual, Dr Lara Briden explains that anti-inflammatory drugs can reduce menstrual flow by up to 50 per cent.

GENTLE EXERCISE

Movement can help lessen cramps, but this is not the time to expect a marathon of yourself (unless marathons are your thing, because you can still kick butt with some planning and careful scaffolding). If you have lower back pain, try yoga poses that will stretch out your glutes and the big muscles in your legs to relieve some of the tightness. Hold each of the poses for a few minutes to really feel the medicine. Child's pose, cat/cow, pigeon pose and downward dog are all good. Do them in bed if you want. Move your hips in a circle, sway, dance, find whatever makes you feel good.

MASSAGE

If you are in a position to go for a massage, do it or consider asking a friend if they want to do period massage swaps with you. Or do it yourself and roll out those pressure points by lying on the floor with a tennis ball in your sore spots. Better yet, invest in a foam roller. I hardly ever leave home without mine and gladly sacrifice shoe space in my suitcase so I can travel with it.

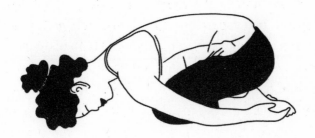

ENDOMETRIOSIS

Most people will experience some kind of period pain, but for one in ten menstruators around the world, the pain can be extreme. Endometriosis is an abundance of tissue similar to the tissue in the endometrium that grows in places other than the endometrial lining (that's the inner lining of the womb; the one that sheds itself when you bleed). This means that there is even more surface area that undergoes removal, renewal and pain production. It can interfere with surrounding tissues in the abdomen area, causing a chronic inflammatory reaction that can lead to problematic scar tissue. The resulting pain can be extremely debilitating.

If you suffer with painful periods, it's likely that your mother and other close female relatives do or did, too, because endo-metriosis has a genetic component. Symptoms can vary wildly, which is why doctors need experience in this area to recognise and properly care for patients with endometriosis. People have had to wait an average of eight years to get diagnosed and treated — a terrible price to pay for menstrual taboo. More research is finally being done so that better treatment options are available and sooner. Early detection and treatment can mean avoidable progression of the condition and can make a huge difference to someone's quality of life. Please don't put up with pain. Know that you are entitled to support.

PREPARiNG TO DO

Here we are, almost at the end of Dream, and like a wall full of jasmine buds you are now about to bloom, big style. Take a moment to look back over the past few days. Did you bleed well? What would you like to do differently next time if you could?

As you come to the end of your bleed, your ideas will start turning into to-do lists. Your body is now gearing up for the next phase in your cycle. Enjoy the return of your mojo but don't overdo it.

You might get flashes of the 'do' feeling. Taste them, roll them around in your mind and notice what exactly you feel compelled to do, and what calls you. Pay attention to anything with a prickly bit of 'should' stuck to it. WHY do you want to do this thing? It can take so long to unlearn the habit of getting on the treadmill and running on autopilot. Just because you start to feel the pull towards doing, doesn't mean you need to. Be protective of your Dream phase.

After a few days of feeling like you've been moving through water, it can feel like the slowness will never end. It will. You can trust that as your oestrogen levels rise you'll be ready to leave the sanctuary of your Dream phase.

You look yourself in the eye at menstruation with love and compassion to welcome all that you are, back into the sanctum of yourself. After many cycles of this, exploring your depths, you'll come to know the way to your heart like the back of your hand.

And now, it's time to DO.

CHAPTER 5

DO

Imagine a queen unfurling from the deepest, most restorative sleep in the Dream cave. She has taken care of herself and allowed her dreams to lie quietly within the most peaceful part of her, and now they are ready to be brought forth. She throws off the duvet, flexes her biceps and does a little spin for good measure. She cares not for holding herself back. The mountain beckons, and she leaves the valley with fire in her belly and a banana in her pocket; she is going up. Today is a good day, and she is ready to DO.

Make way for the 'can-do' queen. Seriously, get out of her way, and quickly, or she'll bowl you over.

It's morning. The sun is shining. I need to . . . DO! All the things! Go for a jog, make wholemeal muesli, finish my project

and plant some kale. Wait . . . I should start a charity. I've got an
incoming egg, people. I NEED TO GET CRACKING!

Welcome to your second phase, an energetic time when your body readies itself to drop a beautiful golden egg. In fact, if you are in this pre-ovulation week right now, I wouldn't be surprised if you are too busy 'doing' to read this.

Imagine a broody bird getting its nest ready for a precious egg: do you think she has time to hang out with her friends, poo-ing on strangers and chatting about who got the fattest worm? No. It's business time; she has a nest to perfect and plans to execute. She's on the clock.

Everything happens a little bit faster now: thinking, walking, talking, making decisions, organising everybody else (often with-out them even noticing; a heartbreaking reality, but who cares right now, you have bigger fish to fry). Wave your wand and move on. Sometimes, just doing is its own reward.

So where does all this energy come from? Your rising hormones, that's where — namely oestrogen and a lick of testosterone (flick back to Chapter 2 if you need a reminder). Last week, while you were bleeding beautifully in your Dream phase, a handful of follicles were waking up and starting to produce oestrogen. Now that you've finished bleeding, it's all systems go. One egg prepares for imminent release by getting plumper and plumper and producing more oestrogen, and your whole body responds as your energy levels rise. You feel stronger and faster. The production of this oestrogen also stimulates sero-tonin, which helps us feel happy and confident — double win. Of your four superpowers, this one — the power to do — is up there for being the most super.

KNOW YOUR
do PHASE

FROM DAY 6ISH TO DAY 13ISH
(WHEN YOUR BLOOD STOPS UNTIL YOU OVULATE)

WHY IS IT HAPPENING?

Your golden egg is plumping up with oestrogen, making you stronger and faster.

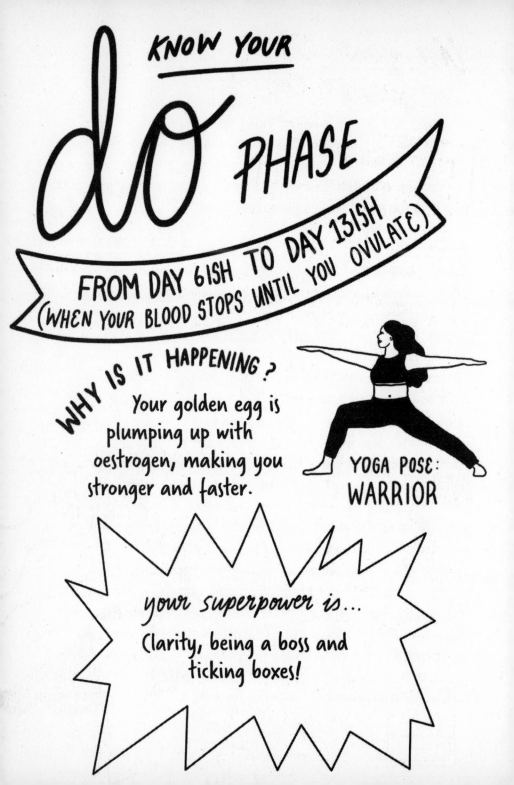

YOGA POSE:
WARRIOR

your superpower is...
Clarity, being a boss and ticking boxes!

Use your Do power to ↘

- get organised and focused
- rise to the challenge
- sow the seeds you saved from the dream phase

!!!CHALLENGES!!!
Feeling frustrated, impatient and overwhelmed with how to use your power.

move your body

#1

yes!

decide on a hero for the month

plan, strategise, keep your eye on the prize

self-care

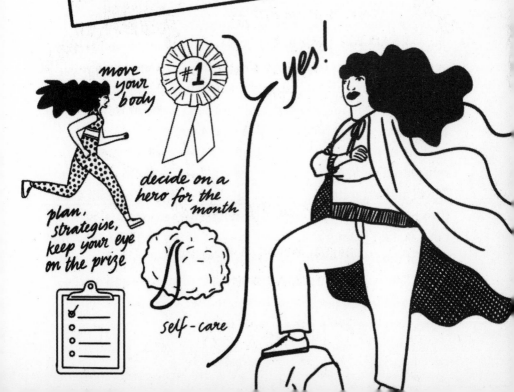

GET TO KNOW YOUR
DO PHASE

By going a little slower and filling up your cup in your Dream phase, you were wisely making energy deposits and building up your balance. Now? It's time to cash in.

The art to nailing life in the Do phase is not blowing it all willy-nilly. Just like in Monopoly, when you've finally passed Go with a fistful of cash, the urge to spend is irrepressible. Behold! Your empire is ready to unfold! But do you really want to buy Old Kent Road and whatever the other brown one is (at my house, we call these 'the poo streets')? Or do you hold out for your big dream: Mayfair and Park Lane, obviously? Of course, you can spend your energy on whatever you want because, with oestrogen on the rise, you can aim for the stars and know you'll make it. You can and you should and you *will*. But what IS your big dream? What do you actually want to grow now? How can you best use this opportunity and this power to Do?

Lots of people feel that moving into the Do phase is just a return to their 'normal': *Finally. I'm not bleeding from the vagina.* It's an understandable cause for celebration in and of itself after the literal drain of your period. And feeling premenstrual is now but a distant memory. Needless to say, this is a common favourite time of the month because everything seems to just happen more easily. The way you respond to the rise in oestrogen and testosterone will be unique to you, but no matter how your hormones affect you, now you are primed for productivity.

Think about what happens in spring, which is the seasonal equivalent to this hormonal phase. The buds on the trees are dormant all winter until the nights shorten and the days get longer and warmer. If the buds emerge too soon, they can suffer during a repeat cold snap and die (similar to the feeling when you rush into Do without a last fantastic long sleep). So they wake up slowly and resume growing before bursting into bloom.

Birds are chirping with joy in the sunshine, and newborn animals are giddy with the excitement of literally just being alive. Life is popping up everywhere, even in cracks in the pavement where little flowering weeds aim their heads for the sun. It feels like this time of growth and possibility will last forever.

This is certainly the phase with the most potential, but to really use this power it needs to be harnessed. Otherwise all of your good ideas end up like newborn lambs headbutting each other at sunset or buds that burst before they're ready to bloom. After sitting by the proverbial fire of menstruation, it's time to get outside and out into the world. When you use this phase to sow the seeds (your deepest dreams) that you saved from last week, you are using your Doing power for maximum effect. Now that your cup is full and you have energy to burn, how on earth will you use it?

When sleeping women wake, mountains will move.
— Chinese proverb

HONOUR THE TRANSITION INTO DO

- Write a list.

- Get out your good undies (and cross your fingers that your period has actually finished).

- Play Tetris or ping pong for peak slaying results.

- Invigorate your room/workspace/wardrobe/the fridge.

- Burn essential oils such as citrus and peppermint to match your elevated mood (or rose if you're feeling tense).

- Organise your clothes in rainbow order.

- Alphabetise the spices in the spice rack, then marvel at your organisational prowess and have everyone else observe and offer praise.

- Get into your activewear with the express intention of being active then do something that makes you red and sweaty while listening to a motivational podcast on double speed (your capacity for comprehension is on point).

- Consider doing some sort of meal preparation for the week ahead so you won't forget to eat nice food while you're kicking ass.

- Decide on your big goal for this month.

- NOW GO AND DO.

DO PHASE ESSENTIALS

💜 Running shoes

💜 Hand weights

💜 Upbeat playlist with empowering anthems to box tick to

💜 Protein balls and nuts

💜 Skipping rope

💜 Positive mantras

💜 A refreshing face mist because you are on *fire* (metaphorically)

TRACKING YOUR DO PHASE

This phase starts cranking up the day after you last bleed, as your oestrogen begins to rise. The transition from Dream to Do might be gradual, with the urge to do and make lists beginning to twitch before your period has even quite finished. Or the shift might be dramatic and sudden. The latter is more common in my experience (provided you are fairly well rested). One morning you're waking up yawning, tired before you've even gotten out of bed, wondering when you'll care deeply about anything ever again, and the next morning? BAM! You burst out of bed wanting to Do like there is no tomorrow. Who knows if there will even be a tomorrow? Who cares? It's now!

When you first start having your period, your body takes a while (years even) to get the hang of regularly releasing eggs. Until it does, your cycles can be up to 45 days long, so you will potentially spend a lot of time here (and also in the lead-up to the Do phase, in kind of a suspended waking Dream/Do state).

With every cycle comes another opportunity to practise ovulation. Eventually, it will occur regularly and your cycle will shorten to about 28–31 days. Even so, this pre-ovulatory Do phase will almost always be longer than the other three phases. And the longer your whole cycle, the longer your Do phase. That means lots of time to try new things, and to persist at learning them and leading others on your merry adventures. Your Do phase will end after the peak oestrogen and testosterone levels cause ovulation about mid-way in your cycle (or later if it's longer than 28 days). Depending on the length of your cycle, you'll spend around nine–twelve days in total 'doing'.

If you have a shorter Do phase, that doesn't mean you do less; if anything, you might actually get more done because this phase is more concentrated and you know you need to make the most of it.

UNLOCKiNG YOUR SUPERPOWER

While the Dream superpower needs some coaxing and convincing that she is welcome, Do just knows she's welcome, so she crashes in with electricity, ready to play like a labrador puppy. This big incoming egg energy is a lot, and sometimes we can get in the way of ourselves.

As well as doing all the nice things you would ordinarily do for yourself, there are few other ways that you can assist your great ascent to fullness. Go, you good thing.

CLEAR YOUR TO-DO LIST

First things first, clear the decks of last month's leftovers before you begin this month's opus. Make a master list of everything that must be done in order of importance/urgency, and then tie your hair back and hit it. If you make a habit of doing this every time your period ends, you'll be less likely to feel guilty about putting things off when you're bleeding.

During this phase, lists are your friends; they relieve your brain of the responsibility of holding it all in, and there is a lot to hold right now. Before your getting-ready-for-bed routine, think about what you'd like to accomplish tomorrow. If you get into bed and still have tasks bouncing around in your 'Tigger brain', get up and write them down. Also, look back over last month's plans to Do and see what needs picking up again or tweaking to fit your direction now.

PAY SOME ATTENTION TO YOUR LOVELY BODY

After hibernating in your heart, it's time to get back into your skin. Honour your exit from the menstrual cave with a full body deep-clean bathing session. Slather on a nourishing face mask and give your body a scrub (you can easily make your own natural products with a quick peruse of the pantry). Hair, nails, kneecaps — the whole nine yards.

In terms of beautification, every hair on your body is an extension of your gorgeous self, but if you do intend to remove some of them using extraction methods, this is the week to do it, when your pain threshold is at its highest. I'm personally a fan of my armpit hair, but I will trim it if it touches my boob (that's when I know). My leg hairs were so long recently that while riding a bike I could feel them blowing in the breeze; it was quite an enjoyable sensation. But I do like a change and the right to choose. Occasionally, I de-fuzz post-period and amass a small pile of hair that could make a tiny jumper. Anyhow, I digress.

FUEL ALL THAT DOING WITH GOOD FOOD

Weirdly, even though your energy is at its highest now and in theory you're firing on all cylinders, your metabolism (your ability to burn energy from food) is now at its slowest. So you just don't need as much fuel right now as you do when you are premenstrual, for instance (when your metabolism is at its highest). Maybe this is nature's way of preparing for a potential pregnancy: by storing up extra energy before ovulation to ensure enough is in the bank if you *were* to conceive.

As always, eat what you feel is good for you. But be aware that if you favour rich and heavy foods now, you might feel a bit blergh and sluggish. And by sluggish I mean bloated (common before ovulation anyway, so we don't want to exacerbate that) and potentially a bit constipated. Not fun if you want to move fast. Enjoy fresh, wholesome food. Greens are especially good.

GET PHYSICAL

Have you ever had the urge to spontaneously change your whole room around and 45 minutes later you've actually done it? You've shifted a roomful of furniture by sitting on the floor and using the brute strength of your mother-loving thighs, and you've got a little sweat moustache and a pink face. As you survey your handiwork you think to yourself, *Heck, I am bloody amazing.* AND IT'S TRUE. Sometimes I throw myself into an exercise class with so much vigour that I am rendered incapacitated for the rest of the week, walking like a cowboy after too many squats. As I said earlier, it's tempting to use all of your Do power at once!

At this time in your cycle you are pumping out oestrogen, which makes you physically faster and stronger. You are so capable now and ready for a challenge. Whether that's on the soccer field or dancing your butt off, this is when you should most delight in feeling physically powerful.

See what you are made of and actually make more of it — I'm talking about your muscles. It's a well-known fact among sports physiologists that this time of the month brings the best opportunity for strength training because oestrogen is 'anabolic', or muscle building. Many women will train harder at this time to make the most of this. You could just carry some baked bean cans while you power walk or do lunges while you're getting dressed.

WATCH YOUR KNEES

If you plan on partaking in any strenuous activity or you play a lot of sport, it's particularly important to warm up in the Do phase of your cycle. Research shows that female athletes are at least three-and-a-half times more likely than males to sustain injuries to their anterior cruciate ligament (ACL), one of the main stabilisers in the knees. You are most at risk if you play pivoting sports such as basketball, netball or soccer, where you're more likely to stop suddenly and land while twisting. Clearly, a woman in her Do phase isn't meant to stop suddenly, if at all.

Studies have shown that this increased risk is related to the way that elevated oestrogen levels affect our tendons. So while knees always need looking after, they especially need it before ovulation. You can also help to prevent these types of injuries by building strength in your core muscles, quads and hamstrings to improve stability while you are leaping and landing.

If you haven't started moving since your period finished, now is the time. It's normal to wake up with a jolt and find to-do lists dancing in your brain, and it's easy to convince yourself that you are too busy for exercise. You aren't, and your body is desperate to move. Sometimes, it's good to feel slouchy or maybe even a bit bored; this feeling often precedes a good idea. But during *this* phase, if you sit around feeling sluggish you won't be feeding the parts of yourself that are hungry for adventure.

Obviously, it's good to get the recommended 30 minutes of aerobic activity a day, but something is always better than nothing. Whether that's ten minutes of yoga or skipping while the kettle boils, just move in whatever way feels good to activate your body and focus your mind.

USE YOUR DO PHASE POWER

How can you do this? However you want, obviously. Wherever it is you want to get to or from, you're more able to see a clear path now. And if you can't, you have the required gumption to hack one out of the wilderness yourself.

This is probably the least sentimental phase in the cycle. You aren't as attached or concerned with how your plans or solutions will impact others, and this is generally a good thing (particularly if you are prone to extreme empathy). If you spent your life in the Dream phase, turning over every potential solution to an issue and considering the ramifications ad nauseum, you'd be trapped in a consideration loop and you'd never get anything done.

Now that you've run any problems through your Dream filter, it's time to sort them out. It's time to act.

In this section, we'll look at how to nurture that little spark of Do so that it turns into a flame that burns bright with purpose.

The most effective way to do it, is to do it.
— *Amelia Earhart (American aviation pioneer)*

DECIDE WHAT YOU WILL GROW NEXT

Look back over any journalling you did in your Dream phase. What was calling your attention at the start of the month? Your growing follicles produce more and more oestrogen the bigger they grow. But now, most of them will degenerate, leaving you with one beautiful ripening egg — I like to think of this as your big project for the month. You might have lots of good ideas about things you want to do, but you can't do them all at once. You did such a good job last week at saying no to non-essential tasks and requests, now you don't need to say yes to everything just because *you can*.

So, with your one grand egg, pick a hero idea and let that be the thing you grow the most this month. It could be building a website, starting a new creative project, applying for a grant, focusing on a health issue or planning a new side hustle. Whatever it is, don't worry about picking the wrong thing; you can always change tack next month or decide on something different. Don't worry about the best place to start. The trick is to just start.

MOBILISE AROUND A HERO GOAL

The magic of the Dream phase comes to fruition as the rest of the entire cycle unfolds, but the Do phase is where most of the work gets done. Set aside some time for planning and scheduling now in order to get this goal into the ground good and proper.

Start by asking yourself three key questions:

1. What are the small parts to this goal that I can tackle now?

2. What are the biggest parts that will take more work?

3. Who can I reach out to for support?

Start by brainstorming a few bullet points to flesh out all of the different components to your hero goal and then embrace whatever organisational process you prefer. Whether it's bullet journalling or using some sort of task-management app or colour-coded mind map, make sure you attach timeframes to each task or groups of tasks.

Use paper, pens, highlighters, stickers, interpretive dance . . . maybe you need to brainstorm with someone else — whatever helps you visualise the logistics of your big picture clearly.

Obviously, it doesn't all need to happen today or in this phase, or even this month, but the planting and the bulk of the planning does. Every time the Do phase rolls around, revisit your goals and see how they're coming along.

Lastly, plan around your actual phases! When you schedule in tasks, think about which phase you will do them most effectively in and — if it's possible to — schedule them in those phases. If something is mentally challenging, tackle it in Do, before ovulation. If it requires connecting with others, asking for help or doing group work, book these sessions during your Give phase, after ovulation, when your Do spark is a bit more manageable and you're able to listen more readily.

If something requires a sharp, critical focus (such as editing, for example), make time for it during Take, when you're premenstrual and quite happy to slash and burn. You might have extra energy now in Do, but it won't be suited to every type of task, so plan where you can to make use of all of your superpowers *when you have them.*

AND ANOTHER THING!

This phase is a good time to tackle any other life maintenance you've been putting off. With your focus face on now, those onerous tasks that you can't see, things like purchasing car insurance, applying for a new passport or booking in for that pap smear your doctor keeps writing to remind you about are less onerous. Good for your life, but also for tidying up your brain. Use it until you lose it!

HARNESS THE POWER OF YOUR BRAIN

Flex your muscles and give yourself a high five because you'd better believe you can do whatever you want now, and should (do whatever you want). Not only is your body primed this week, but your brain is also — actually, it *needs* you to try new things and challenge it while you are primed to prune and myelinate.

Your brain is the last organ in the body to reach maturity. Psychiatrist Dr Daniel J. Siegel, author of *Brainstorm*, explains that from the teenage years until the late twenties, our brains are basically a construction site with two main important jobs to do.

1. Prune

If your childhood years were about growing your brain into a beautiful garden full of synapses (connections between two nerve cells in the brain), then early adulthood is about cutting that growth back, to streamline and tidy it up — to *specialise* your brain. This 'synaptic pruning' coincides with the time in your life when you are finding your passions: what you love and what you definitely do not love. The principle behind pruning is 'use it or lose it'. This is why you should do more of whatever it is you *want* to be good at — dance, soccer, rapping or crochet. Your brain is looking to finetune your synaptic connections, so the wider your range of experiences, the more opportunities you give your brain to develop and specialise in different ways.

2. Myelinate

Once that synaptic pruning has occurred, the next job of the brain under construction is the formation of myelin. Myelin is made of lipids (fats) and proteins (another reason why you need good fats in your diet), and it forms a sheath around connected nerve fibres, which increases the speed with which they can signal each other. You are (literally) getting an upgraded connection.

Whatever you give your attention to and focus on is what you will get better at; it's as simple as that. If you are able to afford it, try new things all the time. If you don't like them, that's okay, just give it a shot and see what you think. Take a class in fencing, football, piano, dance, debating, Japanese. Or teach yourself ukulele, cake decorating, how to trade stocks, permaculture. Don't limit yourself; USE this hyper-connectivity while your maturing brain is thirsty for new experiences, because you will never be able to make the most of them as well as you can *right now*. This is how your passions emerge.

In this phase, you are particularly able: your whole system is geared for going, and you can DO HARD THINGS. Put yourself out there and say yes.

PLAY TO YOUR STRENGTHS AT WORK

After being a bit dreamy last week, during this phase you can dig deep and really Do.

If you've got a project on your plate that needs doing, it will take you less time than it would have last week, so you can be ultra-efficient and super-smug while you Do like the wind. Why are you even still reading this? You're primed for success right now, and you can also use this fervour to start good habits (flossing, for instance) while your motivation is high.

PLAN TO KICK ASS

My friend Odette Mercy (who I told you about back in Dream) is constantly in demand for her voice, her ability to command a whole crowd and for her ideas about direction. She was thrilled to be contacted by a new company in Sydney to help write a musical. 'When can we have you?' they asked. She checked her diary and thought, *Well, here is good, and here is okay and . . .*.

Then she had a brainwave (a womb wave, even): *Hang on a second. If I can choose when to do this very exciting and challenging thing then I choose the DO phase for maximum results.* And she did. She flew over to Sydney when her period finished and spent a week writing a musical and kicking ass. That's how you go with your own flow.

If you are lucky enough to have a presentation, an exam or a big pitch scheduled this week, then do a happy dance because you've already won. You'll find you are able to work more quickly and efficiently under pressure. In fact, you'll thrive on it. Your neurons will be firing together like nobody's business and lighting up like a Christmas tree so this is a good time to solidify your understanding of the concepts at hand, while your brain is at maximum capacity.

If there's a creative project that needs attending to and it's not flowing for you here, see if you can schedule it for a phase better suited to that purpose. Tasks that require you to sit in one spot and think in a more abstract way might feel frustrating to you now because it contradicts the Do superpower, and you do not want to mess with that force.

WING IT (AND NAIL IT)

Planning is important in order to direct energy effectively. However, if you do need to wing it, this is the time of the month when you can really fly by the seat of your pants.

While writing this book, I was at a theatre conference to pitch *My Greatest Period Ever*. I had been home for two days after touring the show in the UK and still felt like my body was catching up with me. While on the plane, I noticed that the date of the pitch would land on Day 11 of my cycle, smack in the middle of my Do phase. *Perfect timing to nail a pitch.*

This meant I could rest on my laurels a bit, deal with my jetlag and be confident that I'd have chutzpah to burn on the day. The morning of the pitch, I washed my hair and warmed my voice up in the shower. I remembered my lucky lipstick just before I walked out to a sea of faces. And you know what? I *did* nail it. I marvelled at how good it felt to rely on my inner powers.

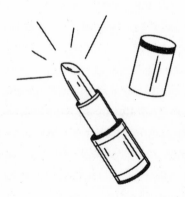

SPEAK UP AND TAKE CHARGE

If you're in a meeting, speak your mind. If you're in class, raise your hand. Think of all the things that need doing in this world: finding a solution for a group project, discovering new ways to generate clean power or just deciding where to get the best kebab at 2 am. We need smart, capable people (like you) who have clear thoughts and can run with them. Raise your hand, raise your voice and get out of your seat. Don't play small.

And while we're at it, let's talk about emailing. Hands up if the time you've spent fretting over your online tone would amount to enough hours to learn a foreign language (puts hand up). If you've been mulling over a few emails during the Dream phase, this is the time to send them. You can still be friendly, but avoid undermining yourself or apologising. Be clear, say what you mean and ask for what you want.

All of this powerful Do energy is a serious force to be reckoned with. Your assertive self emerges now like a panther ready to pounce; she's quick, feisty and not inclined to suffer fools. She doesn't want to know about feelings. She wants to get the thing done.

While everyone else in the room or the group chat is cogitating, you can deftly swoop in with a plan. You might not have the patience to ponder input from the eight other people in the group, but that's precisely *why* you can get things going. It's your turn to be the driver, to lead and to be assertive. You don't need to stomp on other people's ideas, but if something needs doing and you can see how, then speak up. Say, 'I've got this; here's what I think.'

You might not always get unanimous support but you'll probably find most people are relieved that someone is taking control. So take it. Back yourself. If someone calls you bossy, take it as a compliment. If you really believe in what you're doing, this is a good time to fight for it.

The more you practise your power, the more you'll feel able to employ it. You don't need to get arrested, but this part of you needs a chance to grow or it can come and go, unused and unsung, and leave you feeling frustrated and disappointed. Deny your Do power at your peril (and the planet's).

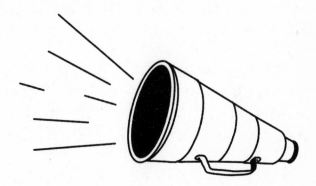

CHALLENGES iN THE DO PHASE

Some people will naturally soar in their Do phase. They'll feel the rise in energy, know exactly what to do with it and wish they could spend their whole lives here. Compared to the challenges you might face in Dream and Take, Do is generally a pretty sweet ride. We're rewarded well for our energy levels, organisational skills and inclination for enthusiasm. That said, there can be a few bumps in the road that hold you back from reaping the full spectrum of Do's benefits.

FEELING OVERWHELMED

Remember that this Do phase is fuelled by high levels of oestrogen in your body, and when you have a lot of oestrogen you can also feel a bit more anxious; it's quite a pushy hormone.

This phase, with its more bombastic, ballsy drive, used to scare the crap out of me. I loved having my period, being all dreamy and letting go and feeling connected to the Earth and nature and everything feeling calm and slow and peaceful and la, la, la. And then whoa, whoa, *WHOA*.

Feeling overwhelmed and searching blindly for your gifts is par for the course when you are 'womaning'. Learning how to use your gifts is something that can and should take a long time, or even a lifetime, to master. That's why being a good learner is an important skill in this phase especially.

Even now, I still find that I feel more anxious during this post-period/pre-ovulation week than at any other time in my cycle. I can feel my cup filling so fast with energy and I have all these lists of things I need to do and I don't know where to start and I can feel the blood pulsing in a spot inside my ear and I feel like a cross between a bull in a china shop (with all of this rising energy) and a deer in the headlights (because what the bleep am I supposed to do with it all?). I call this my 'bull–deer' moment.

Like many girls, I grew up in a culture that rewarded compliance, and where female leadership was maligned as bossiness. Boys weren't called bossy; they were confident, assertive. I would feel a rush of conviction and simultaneously a need to keep a lid on it. It was easier to keep it all in than to risk letting a bit out and losing control of it, like a dam opening its floodgates. I felt unable to contain or direct it.

Now that I know this about myself — that I have a bull–deer wig-out day when oestrogen and testosterone are peaking — I know to expect it, and I also know that it will pass. I treat this bull–deer feeling like a puppy that needs to go on a walk; I tell it where we're going and off we go. Instead of holding it in, I actually use it.

Sometimes feeling overwhelmed by all the things we want and need to do can get in the way of doing anything at all. Rest assured that you don't need to plant the whole farm in one day. If you have children, spending your Do power folding socks and cutting sandwiches into small squares can sometimes make you feel as far away from your 'thing' as if you were in Timbuktu. *Where is my thing? Will I ever have it again?* Don't despair. As with exercise, doing a little bit is far better than doing nothing.

Whether it's signing up for a newsletter, reading it, sending one email or making one call, bit by bit you'll nudge yourself closer and closer to your big goal.

SELF-TALK FOR MANAGING ANXIETY

There is a sense of urgency that comes with this phase. *Am I doing enough?* you might ask yourself. What is 'enough' anyway? Anxiety makes everything feel faster, and when you're already faster during pre-ovulation, you can feel too freaking fast. Slow down for a bit, for a day or an afternoon, and ask yourself if, instead, your anxiety is trying to tell you something. Do you feel out of balance? Are you staying true to your deepest dreams?

Go back to your Dream journalling to feel grounded; when you feel rudderless, remember to use your anchor. Ongoing pressure and anxiety raise your stress hormones, and being in this fight-or-flight state can seriously interfere with a healthy cycle, preventing you from ovulating and missing out on lovely progesterone, which you especially need to soothe anxiety. These simple self-care actions often help me work my way through a bull–deer wig-out, but get extra help if you need it.

- ♥ Breathe deeply and make a sound as you exhale.

- ♥ Do yoga or go for a walk to burn off some of the Do phase intensity.

- ♥ Get vitamin D from the sun to increase your serotonin production (which helps you feel calm and focused).

- ♥ Eat (well) and avoid caffeine. (It's the devil for anxiety.)

- Talk to yourself like a best friend would — out loud with soothing words of encouragement and reassurance. Focus on what is working and dine out on that.

- Make a to-do list on paper to get that stuff out of your head.

- If you're feeling bogged down about how to move your big goal forward, get help and reach out to a mentor. If you don't have one, find them in your next phase when you're primed to connect.

THINKING YOU NEED PERMISSION

Although I always knew I had something big in me, I had no idea what it was or how to get it out. I lacked confidence and doubted that the dreams I desperately wished for would take flight. I frittered my energy away on things that weren't that important to me.

I was pretty good at school, but I moved around a lot, so maybe that made it harder for me to find 'my thing'. And in the absence of finding it, I probably used more of my Do power than I care to admit obsessing over boys (who were mostly oblivious to my romantic musings).

What might I have done differently if I had worried less about making mistakes? What might I have learned about my Do power if I knew my value was so much more than what people thought of me, or how attractive I was to boys?

I tried lots of things after I finished school: nursing, metallurgy . . . getting my truck driver's licence. I thought *maybe* I could sing. Now I realise I was waiting for someone to give me permission: permission to try, to be bad at something or even excellent at it.

You know something?

You don't need permission.

Please say that in your head and out loud over and over until you believe it. *You don't need permission* to do anything that you want and, most of all, you don't need permission to be a bit crap or quite crap at something. Unless you have a freakish talent, you'll probably be a bit crap whenever you start something new (I mean, you could be extremely crap). But that's OKAY!

Think back to when you first started learning anything difficult, riding a bike for example. Imagine if when you'd hopped on the first time and then fell off, your parents had said to you, 'Well, Emily, you clearly don't have what it takes. Stick to crayons.'

Anything worth doing takes effort. We all know that. And if you fail, really, who cares? You have a right to fail, to stuff up and make a big fat mess. And the longer you stick at 'the thing', the better you will get. There are plenty of people doing things that they aren't brilliant at, yet. Maybe they never will be, but they do those things because it feels good to do them and because they want to. And those are the only reasons you need; permission is not required.

It used to be, though. It's only in recent history that opportunities have opened up for women to be excellent in areas that were traditionally male-dominated. Generations of women were encouraged to pursue more 'feminine' professions such as nursing or teaching (if they were lucky to have a profession at all) instead of exploring their unique talents to their fullest capacity. Thank goodness things have changed.

But have they changed *enough*?

Currently, the number of girls taking up science, technology, engineering and mathematics (aka STEM subjects) at school in Australia is lower than ever. Why? A recent study revealed that this wasn't because girls don't like those subjects or because they aren't actually good at them, but rather because boys have a greater sense of belief in their own abilities than girls do. It seems we're still dealing with the cultural hangover of being told that we can't do things. Screw that. Please, please, if not for you then for your grandmother, have a go at everything and anything you want to. Take a bite and see if you like the taste.

Listen to that little voice in your head that whispers, *Go on, have a try. You can do it*. Then give it a megaphone. Dial it up to 11. This is your deep inner knowing, and after a good rest in the Dream phase, she is ready to be seen. 'Look at me. Watch me,' she says. 'I can do this.' She's ready to strut her stuff, so don't hold her back. Let her off the chain and trust her. Grant yourself permission.

Once you find your 'thing', you'll discover that having it gives you somewhere to aim your Do power. And then not only will you get better at your thing, but it will also start to feel more and more natural to be good at *all* things. When you strengthen all of those emotional muscles, eventually your body and mind come to know the drill. *Ah*, you'll whisper to yourself, *this is how we do it*.

HOW i FINALLY GAVE
MYSELF PERMISSION

As a kid, I remember singing along to opera in the bath or while playing in the garden. I didn't know or care if I was good at it, it just felt normal. I loved singing.

In Year 3 while we were learning how to sing harmonies for 'Three Blind Mice', our music teacher said, 'Girls on this side singing high and boys on that side singing low'. I tried singing the high notes, but I didn't like it so I sang the low bits instead and it felt good (turns out my voice is deeper). The teacher corrected me, though, and instructed me not to sing the 'boys' parts'.

I'm sure she meant no harm, but at eight years old I went from honestly believing that I could sing opera (which I now know takes decades to perfect) to feeling that I couldn't even sing 'Three Blind Mice' because I couldn't sing like a girl. After that, I only sang to myself.

Finally, at eighteen, I thought that maybe I could sing. After listening to the singer in my boyfriend's heavy metal band scream so much his neck veins popped out, I was sure that I was definitely maybe as good or even better than him. But where to start? What to do? I found an ad for a choir in the community paper and made a cautious plan to join. When I arrived at the audition, the choirmaster opened his front door and sighed as he looked me up and down. 'Come in, stand by the organ please.'

Whatever I did in that audition was evidently not what he was after because he said that I wasn't suitable for the choir. I thanked him for his time, and as I drove home, I reasoned that while I thought I *might* have been able to sing, he was clearly an 'expert who knew'. So obviously I couldn't. What next? I enrolled in a biomedical science degree, and it would be almost ten years before I really started singing again.

The great thing about your 'thing' is that it will find a way out eventually. At twenty-six, I had a baby. How I loved (and still love) him. I was so happy tending to his every need. Eventually, when he was nine months old and starting to move around on his own, I realised with a jolt that I didn't need the permission of that teacher or an ancient choirmaster to sing. *If I can grow a baby inside of me*, I thought, *I'm pretty sure I can do whatever I want.*

So I gave myself permission. I auditioned to be the lead singer in a band and I got in. I taught myself how to play a baritone ukulele while my little boy pottered in the dirt with his trucks and dolls. I wrote songs and started doing shows with my band. When I couldn't get a babysitter, I'd take my son with me. I'd breastfeed him and then buckle him into his car seat, driving around with classical music and the heater on until he fell sound asleep. I'd arrive at the venue and ask a friend or my sister to sit with him while he slept, so I could sing for 45 minutes. Then I'd drive home and get into bed with him, exhausted and elated.

If you want to do something, it's because you should. The secret to your superpower is to keep using it. Answer an ad or write your own. And if it doesn't work out? Who cares. Make another plan and try again. This little flame in you will grow to be a fire if you tend to it for long enough.

YOU DON'T FEEL LIKE DOING

If it feels like your fire is more of a smoking pile of ash and your Do power is nowhere to be seen, maybe you need a little bit more rest.

You stop bleeding after your Dream phase, then wait, ready for the lift to take you up into Do and then, and then . . . it doesn't come. You *still* feel tired. You don't feel motivated and, to make matters worse, you were *expecting* to feel energetic so now you feel disappointed that you feel low. And you have a to-do list as long as your arm.

The more you can slow down and rest in your Dream phase, the more energy you'll have in this one. However, it can often feel like the universe is conspiring to make resting extremely difficult or near on impossible. An afternoon with my sister and her two small children reminds me that sometimes self-care is having a shower alone and rubbing your eyes for a full minute as a treat.

It's never too late (or too early for that matter) to rest. Give yourself a break, pass your to-do list to someone else if possible and rewind back to deep rest before you try again. Maybe you need to *be* a bit longer before you *do*.

RELATIONSHIPS

If you had a good Dream phase and emerged from hibernation ready to Do with not a moment to lose, it can feel like everybody else around you is frustratingly *S L O W*.

That's because they are. As you hurtle closer to ovulation and your Give phase, you basically become superhuman in terms of your life/speed capacity. You are built for tackling goal-orientated tasks at this juncture, and people's feelings can seem like an unbearable deviation from the job at hand.

Sometimes, when I'm explaining something to someone, having to stand there and wait for what feels like an eternity while they compute my big, fabulous idea is excruciating. 'CATCH *UP*!' you want to bark, because you are on fire and your body knows that this won't last forever. Next week you'll be more inclined to share more slowly. Now? Not so much.

Significant relationships might go on the backburner a bit during Do because you are mentally and physically on the move (my desire to snuggle in bed in the morning takes a serious nose-dive). If you've been meaning to do some mending in a relationship, you may not get the desired result if you take a crack at that now. Save those chats for next week, when you are more able to feel deeper empathy and the desire to connect.

BURNOUT AND FINDING BALANCE

Many people love this phase the most and would happily live here all month because this is the part of us that experiences the most 'success' for our achievements. It's easy to see how this phase can feel like the 'real' you, and the other parts of our cycle can get edged out. But, like Eloise (who you'll meet on the next page) discovered, it's a tough gig to keep up all month, and the real take-home message here is balance.

EVERY BODY HAS A LIMIT

Meet Eloise, a former elite rower who trained for up to six hours a day, every day, for six years. She felt most at home in the Do phase, where she was kicking ass and feeling strong.

Eloise loved to row and she loved to compete. Every day she would weigh herself ahead of the weekly race to qualify for her weight division. She thrived under the pressure; the only thing getting in her way was her period. To Eloise, having a period was not just a burden but also incredibly debilitating thanks to the symptoms: chronic migraines that sometimes made her pass out from pain, convulsing shakes and vomiting. Eloise came to rely heavily on painkillers. As she puts it: 'Training for a sport I loved and having a period at the same time was a nightmare.'

Eventually, her passion for rowing drove her body into the ground. Her gut health was a mess because of the painkillers, and her period caused her excruciating pain three days a month. Despite the pain, her periods were actually getting lighter. Blood tests revealed an overload of testosterone, which Eloise now attributes to her gruelling schedule: 'I didn't have enough fat on my body and I was in a state of permanent stress. Cycle health wasn't spoken about.'

It was her older brother who started searching for answers after seeing her in pain. Eventually, she realised the impact of pushing too hard, for too long. Eloise had been stuck in the Do phase without giving her body time to rest.

When her time for competitive rowing came to an end, she was devastated but chose to use the change as a positive event and get to the bottom of why her fading period had become so debilitating. She started healing simply, by paying attention to how she felt and slowing down even more during her period. Gradually, her pain began to improve.

She spent two years exploring ways to care for her cycle and connect with it. After seeing a naturopath, osteopath and acupuncturist, and experimenting with abdominal massage, yoni steaming and lots of rest, Eloise says the difference is incredible. 'I'm so happy now, and in disbelief that a period can feel this great. I've literally dreamed of pain-free periods for years and this month has been a dream come true.'

Looking back, Eloise says, 'I spent a long time kind of hating that I was a girl.' As someone who naturally thrived in the Do phase, she came to love the other parts of her cycle and saw that she also needed rest and balance in order to have a *sustainable* Do power.

Working on self-love was a big part of her healing. But the single most helpful thing has been learning how to work with, and appreciate, the beauty and incredible nature of the female cycle. Now she loves herself best all month long.

Today, Eloise is a personal trainer for young, competitive elite female athletes. She's a passionate advocate for menstrual cycle awareness, and teaches the young women she trains to use their cycles to their advantage. With her help, those young women won't have to fight against their natural rhythms the way she did.

THE DISTANT DO-ER

A family I'm close with has been cycle savvy for about three years now. Their daughter, Sophie, is fourteen. She lives with her mum, younger brother and sister, and stepdad, Will.

Will tells me that understanding and appreciating the two cycles happening in his household has 'pretty much saved my marriage as well as my relationship with my teenage stepdaughter'.

Sophie is smart, funny and partial to an Olympic-grade eye roll, and Will now has some valuable insights about her. He notices that they enjoy more family time together listening to music when she has her period.

Of her premenstrual phrase, he lovingly says, 'It's a more intense time, sure, but I'm glad to be there for her.'

Turns out the hardest time for Will to connect with Sophie is when she's in her Do phase. But now, rather than thinking, *How hard is it to say good morning?*, he realises what's really going on: *Oh, we're in the Do phase. No one else exists, she's on a mission.*

He understands that he needs to be patient when Sophie is sitting on a goldmine of possibilities. He respects that she is driven to do certain things RIGHT NOW, and he gives her the space to do them. He knows that next week will be a different story (all going to plan, of course).

COMPARISON
(AKA THE THIEF OF JOY)

The hit of testosterone before ovulation can make you feel more aggressive, driven and goal-orientated — in the wild, this is when female animals compete for a mate.

Enjoy feeling fierce and powerful and driven to win whatever it is you have your sights set on, but watch out for feelings of insecurity, or comparing yourself. Instead of seeing someone else and thinking, *They are so much more fabulous than me. I will never be that fabulous/that type of fabulous.* Think to yourself, *Holy wow. She is fabulous. How fabulous is she? Go HER.*

Fabulousness is an infinite resource. The more comfortable you are seeing it in others, the more you will see it and celebrate it in yourself.

In her book *Fight Like a Girl*, Clementine Ford reminds us to actively undo the old Disney ideal, where a woman's currency is dependent on her perceived attractiveness to a man. When women are portrayed like this, as props in movies, their self-worth is in the hands of another and that's a bloody lie.

Not only does this rob us of genuine, authentic connections with the opposite sex, but it also denies us the powerful, joyous bonds to be had with other girls because we are set up to compete against each other for the finite resource of someone else's attention. We are so much more than whether or not we are liked. Other women are your allies, and they need you to be theirs, too.

PREPARING TO GIVE

It's time to look forward to opening up and celebrating your victories.

If Do was about blooming, then Give is about picking the fruit (and sharing it). But, of course, you only get to harvest what you sow. So when your power to Do presents herself in front of you — gleaming, glinting like Athena, goddess of wisdom and war — and hands you a silver platter and a quest destined just for you, step up to the challenge. It's yours for the taking.

As you get closer to the Give phase, think about who you can bring in to your latest scheme or idea, or who can help you with your hero goal. Who do you want to connect with? Who will inspire you and fuel your fire? Who do you want to have a picnic under a tree with? Plan for connecting next week, and include time for some heart-to-hearts with your nearest and dearest.

From here, things slow down a smidge and soften. Get ready to ease into Give.

Day 13 Dream Journal

I dreamed I was in a car. It was black, old and American, and so cool. The window was down, wind in my hair, then the car just stopped. I hopped out and tried to keep it moving with one hand on the steering wheel, but it was heavy and hard work. The lights ahead went amber. I started to panic. What if I got caught in the middle? Then I thought, stuff it. The car was aimed in the right direction, I could just get behind it and push! So I did. It was easier than I'd imagined.

CHAPTER 6

GIVE

Imagine a queen who's arrived at the summit of a mountain, Peak Fabulous. Windswept and glorious, she looks out over the valley behind her, mightily satisfied with her progress. The air is sweet, she takes in a lungful and her skin glistens in the sunlight. *I did it*, she thinks, hand on her hip. In the distance she sees her friends approaching, eager to delight in her bounty and her generous spirit. It's time to celebrate. It's time to say, 'Yes! Absolutely yes to everything! All of the things!' More than ever, it feels like she is in exactly the right place at exactly the right time. She knows that right now her capacity for connection is peaking. She knows it's time to Give. She walks towards them with her arms open wide.

Your Give phase begins at ovulation and marks the start of the second — luteal — half of your cycle. You've just laid one of your precious eggs, and you are all about it. You're still riding high on the ass-kicking capabilities of Do, but there's also a softness and a smoothness, making you feel like you have the world on a string. If that isn't a cause for a celebration, I don't know what is.

This phase is a magic, juicy time; it's so good, in fact, that it can be a little hard to let go of. It helps if you pace this big egg energy by saving a secret stash of it away to help you get through the following phase (Take), when you'll head back down Peak Fabulous, back to that cosy cave. But that's all ahead of you, light years away. Swing while you're winning, baby. Time to step up, step out and be seen in the world for the magnificent being you truly are.

You have so much more now — more hormones flowing through your body than at any other time in the cycle, and more to give to those around you. It's time to enjoy the fruits of your labour as the seeds you planted last week in your Do phase come to fullness. With a cup that's overflowing, you are the epitome of extra, and naturally, people are drawn to share in the loveliness of your golden egg afterglow. Honestly, why wouldn't they be?

You might feel pretty delicious (without perhaps knowing that you've just ovulated), or this phase might run on from the Do phase without you noticing anything hugely different until it grinds to a halt as you arrive in the Take phase feeling pre-menstrual. *Gah! What happened? Where am I?* When the Give phase comes to an end, it can be a rude shock, but the more you learn about ovulation and how to notice the signs of it in your body, the more you will see the connection to how it makes you feel (and be able to say goodbye to it).

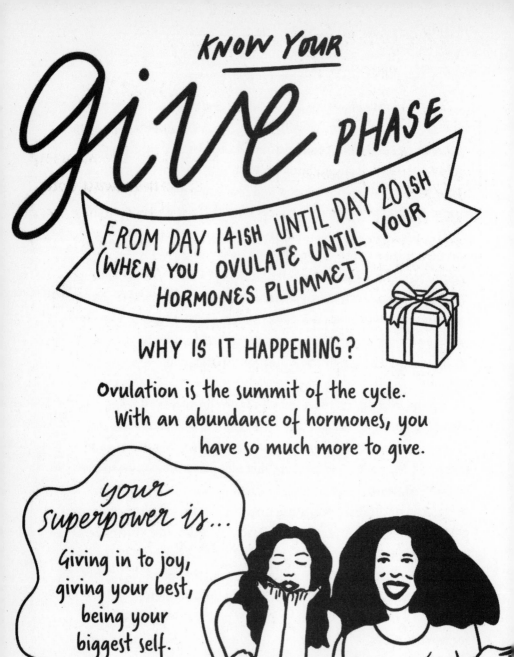

KNOW YOUR

give PHASE

FROM DAY 14ISH UNTIL DAY 20ISH (WHEN YOU OVULATE UNTIL YOUR HORMONES PLUMMET)

WHY IS IT HAPPENING?

Ovulation is the summit of the cycle.
With an abundance of hormones, you
have so much more to give.

your
superpower is...

Giving in to joy,
giving your best,
being your
biggest self.

Use your Give power to

- launch your hero dreams
- enjoy your gorgeous body
- give back
- express gratitude
- reach out and give to those with less

!!!CHALLENGES!!!
Giving away too much, boundaries, frittering away your 'give' energy where it can't grow.

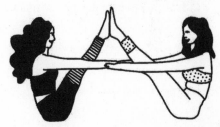

YOGA POSE : PARTNER

yes!

thank you, with love.
pre-write cards or buy gifts for weeks to come

have difficult conversations/ heart-to-hearts

buy yourself some flowers

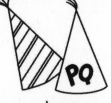
PO
plan a party!

call someone and tell them you love them

offer to cook for your friends, baby-sit their kids etc.

GET TO KNOW
YOUR GIVE PHASE

Ever found yourself walking down a street and feeling compelled to tell random strangers how utterly beautiful they are? That's a classic Give move. The transition into Give is such a sweet spot in the cycle: you see the world through rose-tinted glasses and that rosy glow is reflected right back at you. You are full of potential, in the prime of your summer and at your most fabulous. The job of this phase is to seek out the joyous pockets of life and milk them for all they're worth.

CELEBRATE YOUR FABULOUS SELF

Remember when you were a toddler? When you thought that the world revolved around you and that you looked fabulous in only a pair of knickers and gumboots? (Newsflash, you still do.)

This phase harks back to that time and that exact feeling. At no other point in the cycle will you feel as much sublime queen-liness as you do right now, and this feeling bolsters you through many difficulties like a magic carpet.

Perhaps you catch your reflection in the window, enjoy the sound of your own singing voice, marvel at your winning way with a little baby or feel that all of your friends just love you to bits. (Where is the red carpet already?) Revel in this feeling for as long as you can, and rub it all over yourself like a rich, luxurious moisturiser because you *need* it. It's so good for you. Your body gives you just enough to last until next month, so use every last drop.

If you've caught yourself feeling pretty damn pleased with yourself and then questioned it, or doubted that your 'deserv-ability' level is adequate, stop that as quickly as you can. Don't ever poke a hole in your own fantastic bubble. Appreciation and self-love are the most important tools you can ever cultivate, and this phase is *when* you cultivate them. Life isn't always easy, and when it isn't you can draw from this bank of loving your fine self and it will stand you in good stead for those times when you take a few knocks.

So take the compliments and/or give them freely to yourself. You are not fluking this feel-good feeling, it's a real, true thing and you can rely on it to be there for you month after month. Get used to it.

Now that you are literally full of yourself, this is the time in your cycle where you are least likely to give a shit about what anyone else thinks, especially about your body and your appear-ance. Puff yourself up like a peacock, and feel pride in the face of retail industries based on cultivating insecurity. There's a lot of money to be made by telling women that we need enhanc-ing and that our bodies are 'projects' with 'problem areas'. But not today and not from you; you are perfect the way you are. Especially now.

This is your chance to go to a party in full fancy dress and then decide the next morning, with your make-up still looking good, to live life a little bit more fancy. Dial. It. Up. Dive into your self-expression and try something new: electric-blue eye shadow, hot rollers or statement brows (but do be aware that if you feel inspired to commit to a hairstyle, your future PMS-self might hate you for it). Even if you're working from home, get dressed to meet the world and smell the flowers. Notice the birds and the beautiful sky, and if it feels like it was all put there for you to enjoy, that's because IT WAS! Take a selfie in case you need reminding next week of how bloody gorgeous you are — especially in knickers and gumboots.

HONOUR THE TRANSITION INTO GIVE

- Smile at yourself in the mirror until it stops feeling weird. Sing yourself a little song if necessary.

- Call your grandmother or anyone you love and sing. 'I just called to say I looove you . . .' (No, I haven't been drinking, Mum. Just ovulating.)

- Reach out and ask for help on your big dream and get some guidance from a mentor.

- Explore more self-pleasure.

- Write yourself a love letter. (You may like to revisit this during your Take phase when/if you feel self-critical.)

- Buy a bunch of roses and hand them out to friends, colleagues, maybe even a stranger, or find some other way to spread your sparkle as an act of community service.

- Buy a fabulous new lipstick colour.

- ♥ Give yourself a facial. Give someone else a facial.

- ♥ Plan a gathering or a party to celebrate for no particular reason (we all know the real reason though).

- ♥ Think BIG and enjoy feeling extra.

- ♥ Keep some time free for spontaneity.

GIVE PHASE ESSENTIALS

- ♥ Time: for spending with friends and people you love or for getting your eyeliner perfectly symmetrical on both eyes

- ♥ Clothes that make you feel fabulous

- ♥ Parties or plans to get excited about

- ♥ A lipstick in every pocket

- ♥ A digital thermometer that will give you a reading to two decimal places

- ♥ Celebratory playlist

TRACKING YOUR GIVE PHASE

When your period arrives (in the absence of pregnancy), you can assume ovulation has occurred around 14 days prior. With this in mind, you can predict your approximate ovulation window by simply subtracting 14 days from your average total cycle length. (You can work this out by tracking three months or more of cycles, then working out your average cycle based on that.)

It's normal to fluctuate by a few days (particularly if you are under more stress).

If you are at a stage in your life when your immediate plans do not include pregnancy, this chapter is still very much for you. Even if you never intend to have children, if you were born with a cycle then understanding your fertility is important for your overall health. Yes, your egg is capable of contributing to a pregnancy, but you can also use this phase to birth ideas, projects, relationships and the best parts of yourself, not just babies. You don't need to monitor all or any of these changes to be 'womaning' properly, just know they exist, and that noticing them is a useful way to connect with this part of your cycle — and, in doing so, to connect more deeply with your life.

For a more precise indication of ovulatory evidence, pay attention to these physical signs:

1. Cervical position

Recall your cervix, the gateway between your vagina and your womb. For many of us, a cervix is simply what necessitates the need for a regular pap smear; we associate its existence with the prevention of ill health (and possibly a cold speculum). I previously considered the cervix in isolation and imagined it through the doctor's perspective: pink, vulnerable and slightly indignant when exposed to the harsh light of day. I certainly didn't feel connected to it. Now I see it as another part of my body to be reclaimed and celebrated for its role in the cycle.

The Latin meaning of the word cervix is 'the womb's neck'. And at around 2–3 centimetres long, comprised of muscular tissue and an inner mucosal layer, your cervix forms the lower portion of your womb and acts as a portal between your outer world and your innermost one. By changing shape and producing different fluids, your cervix controls what comes into it and when or how that object may leave. We'll get to those all-important fluids later, but for now, consider how it feels.

Checking your cervical position takes some practise, but it is a useful tool for knowing when ovulation is near and when it has occurred. Here's why: if you were to feel your cervix every day by inserting a finger into your vagina, you would become an expert on your cervix and come to know that, for most of the month, your cervix is sort of doughnut shaped with a taught consistency and a closed opening. In the days preceding ovulation, it's a different story. The cervix rises higher, is fleshier to the touch and its narrow canal is wider. Yes, the evolutionary function of this is so the cervix can welcome in any visiting sperm, but I also like to think of this as the time when you are ushering in *all* types of life; this is a time when you are literally more open.

Feel for yourself. And while you're up there, you'll also notice . . .

2. Slippery, stretchy cervical fluid

Cervical mucus, discharge or fluid: these words do little to herald the magic of this time and, taken on their own, they can seem quite abstract. Mucus doesn't exactly conjure up magic; if anything, it's more commonly associated with the presence of infection. Perhaps instead, we can call it ovulatory *elixir*. Its presence is the most recognisable sign of an imminent egg debut.

After your period finishes, throughout the Do phase, you'll have mostly dry days. But, as the chosen ovarian follicles mature and produce more oestrogen, specialised oestrogen-sensitive cells within the cervix will heed the call for celebration and respond by making the fluid. This fluid happens to aid the passage of potentially available sperm through the cervix towards your soon-to-be-released egg. Without it, sperm would die of exhaustion; in the slightly acidic vaginal cavity, sperm are lucky if they survive for a few hours, but in the presence of this magical elixir, sperm swim on into the womb, welcomed, nourished and prepared to party for up to five days while they anticipate ovulation: 'Now? Now? How about now?'

'When I'm good and ready', replies the egg. She hurries for no one.

You'll notice this life-saving fluid on your underwear, maybe when you wipe yourself after peeing or if you insert half a finger into your vagina on the right day. It feels slippery and stretchable between two fingers — like egg white (I say 'like' egg white but that's exactly what it is. Funny that we are more familiar with the egg of a chicken than our own). Make a note of when this happens in your cycle because the more familiar you are with your different kinds of fluid, the more easily able you will be to detect impending ovulation as well as anything out of the ordinary. Some people make more and some people make less. You'll come to know what is normal for you.

Once progesterone levels rise after the formation of the *corpus luteum* (which we spoke about in Chapter 2), your cervix ceases production. Any passing sperm have now well and truly missed the boat, and their survival will no longer be assisted. That is, until next time . . .

3. **A twinge in your ovary**

Just before, during or after ovulation, you might notice a pang on one side of your lower abdomen as the follicle ruptures to release the ripest egg. The technical term for this is *mittelschmerz*, which is German for 'middle pain' (because ovulation occurs around the middle of your cycle). It can be a small, sharp pain as the follicle bursts or more of a dull, pressurised ache caused by the release of the fluid that the egg floats around in. It shouldn't last for too long or be unbearable, so if it is, speak to a doctor because this is a sign of something worth investigating, such as ovarian cysts.

4. **Basal body temperature (BBT)**

If taking your temperature sounds boring or unnecessary because your cycle is very regular, or you just can't think of anything worse, don't worry about it. But if you want to know when your Give phase has commenced or when you are at your most fertile, then taking your daily temperature can yield useful information.

Once you have ovulated, the production of progesterone raises your temperature slightly by an average of around 0.4 degrees Celsius. (This can explain why your fingers might feel a bit puffy and your rings tighter.) A few months of

collecting this information will enable you to calculate the average day *before* the temperature increase (which is when you ovulated).

To track your temperature, use a digital thermometer under your tongue at around the same time every morning and either record it somewhere or just note the day it peaks. It's important to do this after at least five hours of sleep, before you get up — make it the first thing you do, before your temperature rises in response to any activity.

Tracking your temperature can also be particularly useful if your cycle length is prone to changing (which is common). For instance, I check my temperature every morning on the days after my period then when it spikes I know I ovulated the day before and I *also* know that my period will come 14(ish) days later. I usually ovulate on Day 16, but it's not uncommon for it to happen on Day 13, 14, 15 or sometimes even 17. Your temperature will be able to confirm if you are ovulating or not while using a hormonal IUD.

It's difficult to say *exactly* when the Give phase ends without doing blood tests to detect the drop in progesterone and oestrogen levels. The simple answer is that it's over when you don't feel like giving anymore and that the 'sweet spot' has moved on to something else entirely. It might be subtle or extreme, and it can change from month to month. After a few months, you'll know when you can expect to move into your Give phase (which will help you to use it wisely), and knowing when it will end will help make the move into Take a little smoother.

UNLOCKiNG YOUR SUPERPOWER

As you will soon see, I am a massive fan of spending this Giving part of myself on those I love — that's why I call it the Give phase. Why am I even here if not to love and be loved in return? However, remember that your dearest and oldest friend is yourself.

Recently, my Give phase coincided with a weekend that my husband was going to be away. *Hmm*, I thought, *all this love in the tank and no plans to spend it on anybody.* I immediately started planning but then wondered, *When was the last time I spent this good juju on myself?* Spending time alone in each of your phases deepens your relationship with that part of yourself, and this phase offers a golden opportunity to treat yourself like you would your favourite friend, as a superstar. After all, you and your body worked extra hard last week in Do and this is the time to reward yourself. Speaking of which . . .

SELF-CARE IN THIS PHASE

Last week in your Do phase your energy was rising. At ovulation you are practically superhuman, so make the most of this stamina while you have it. Stay hydrated and fuel your body with good food in much the same way you did in the Do phase; hormones actually 'stick' to fibrous vegetables, that's how we clear them, so ramping up the vegies will support your body to process your surging hormones.

Moving your body now will pave the way for a smoother Take phase; you'll feel less pent-up and crunchy when your hormone levels do fall. Exercise might not feel like a top priority, especially if you find an opportunity to connect with someone instead, but you must move. Opportunities for connection will sprout like weeds in the pavement, so don't let that stop you from this aspect of self-care. Do both. Include more team sports or social exercising such as soccer or playing frisbee in the park. Go for a power walk with a friend, or dance in your living room with your family until you get hot and sweaty. Just move because you can.

YOU DO YOU

This is the time of the month when you can and should feel absolutely divine inside and out. You have just laid an egg after all; you're a goddess with life emanating from every gorgeous pore. Behold the hotness. It can be intense, and you might even find yourself momentarily aching for someone quite unexpected. If you are bereft of a beholder, it can be agonising. *Lustrations*, a high school friend and I named these feelings.

Hold yourself and fan your own flames. This powerful part of you is rightfully yours to enjoy. Take time to explore your entire body on your own terms and find out what pleases you. There are no rules, no wrong ways to be sensual — only maps to be learned and re-learned, off by heart. And it does take some learning to find your shortcuts (or the loveliest long way home), but the best person to teach you is you. Treat yourself like a treasured lover so that you know what it's like to feel this good, no matter who you're with.

Think about whatever you want and touch yourself however you like. Get a mirror and *see* what it feels like to feel this good. Focus on nothing else except the pursuit of your own pleasure, and fall in love with every curve, every crevice, every fold and every shade of yourself. You are the queen of your country.

Sexual pleasure and orgasms release relaxing hormones that help us sleep, deal with stress, and make us feel happy. Also, a good relationship with your sexuality sets you up to enjoy better sexual partnerships.

The UK's National Health Service (NHS) imagined this, too. A campaign informed by sex positive principles was introduced to encourage masturbation in young people so they could be more informed about their own pleasure before beginning sexual relationships with others. They wondered if encouraging masturbation and pleasure would mean young people would not only enjoy their bodies more, but also feel more inclined to have sex only when they were confident that they wanted to. Makes sense.

In Australia, it looks like we need some more encouragement in that department, too. A study of 20,000 people aged between sixteen and sixty-nine found that women were 50 per cent less likely to regularly masturbate than men (or at least to feel comfortable enough about reporting it). Maybe this statistic will even out as women's sexuality is portrayed more positively.

Up until recently, most mainstream (i.e. funded) pop culture was made by men, with women routinely depicted as accessories. I spent much of my movie watching in high school recoiling from movies that failed the Bechdel test (which simply asks if the media in question has two or more named female characters who engage in a conversation about something besides men). Porn, which is also predominantly made by men for a male audience, is more common now. Women's pleasure is routinely depicted as a performance that is secondary to successfully satisfying a male partner. Looking into his eyes is enough to drive her wild with desire and make her come after a few manly thrusts. This tired stereotype doesn't work for most women, who are more interesting and diverse. I would argue that it doesn't work for most men either; they also want more than disconnected goal-orientated sex. Write your own script. If you feel like you are an extra in someone else's movie and you don't like it, talk to them.

The porn industry has a lot to answer for because back when magazines were the most common medium, the gauge for how explicit the content was (i.e. women's bodies) was determined by how visible the labia was. If you could see a woman's labia minora (the inner lips), the image was deemed more explicit and subjected to tighter regulations. The solution: Photoshop out the offending labia minora (oof). Rub, rub with the electronic eraser and . . . problem solved! The real problem then was that millions, mainly men, came to see those (very normal) protruding inner lips as an anomaly. This drove a trend to surgically modify the sensitive inner lips so that they were invisible.

Labiaplasty is the fastest-growing cosmetic procedure in Australia, with the most commonly requested one being 'the Barbie'. Last time I checked, she didn't even have genitals. You already have a designer vagina, so enjoy every bit of it. I say 'designer vagina' because that was plastered on the window signage for a cosmetic surgery near me, and every time I drove past it I mentally hurled a rock through the glass. Your vagina refers to the stretchy passage inside of you. What you can see from the outside — your labia majora, labia minora and clitoris — is what we lovingly call your vulva, and if someone tries to tell you that any part of your exquisite anatomy is anything other than exquisite, do not entertain any part of this lunacy.

Viva your vulva.

HORMONAL CONTRACEPTION AND OVULATION

At twenty-five, I decided that I was ready to have a child with my partner after dating for six weeks. Yes, I know that is ridiculous, and I suppose I knew it at the time, but what can I say? I was ready. I was almost a qualified teacher, I was in love at the most fertile time in my life and the pull was undeniable. I took folate and got pregnant the next month, and I'm forever grateful that we followed our hearts and made our son exactly when we did (particularly as conceiving 15 years later has not been as easy). And this little story provides a handy segue to the elephant in the room: using your eggs for babies. Or not.

There are only a few times in your life, if you so choose, that you will spend your egg on making an actual person. For every other time, you consider how you'll avoid it perhaps with contraception.

Men are fertile every single day of the year, yet women bear most of the reproductive responsibility even though we're only fertile for about five days of the month. There are many methods available (that have barely improved since their invention) and discussing each of them is beyond the scope of this book; suffice to say that hormonal contraceptives (HC) almost always result in the disruption of our natural hormonal cycle.

Having access to information and contraception services is considered a universal human right for teenagers and women, and fundamental to gender equality, though you might rightly feel as though you are choosing the least-crap option. As a teenager, I was eager to exercise this right as soon as I knew that I wanted to have sex.

I told my dad I needed to see a doctor because of an ingrown toenail, but once I was with the doctor, I confessed that what I really needed was to go on the pill. She eyed me up and down, noted that I wasn't yet sixteen and asked if I would be prepared to talk to my parents. When I said no, she reluctantly deemed me responsible enough to make a mature decision and wrote me a prescription. She didn't mention that by taking the pill I would cease to ovulate. I didn't understand how important ovulation was or that I needed it in order to make my own hormones.

As per the tiny print on the insert, I experienced some common side effects: weight gain, headaches, fluid retention, and pimples of a volcanic magnitude. To top it all off, I felt flat and less interested in sex anyway. This reduction in sexual desire is well-documented and ironic given most people take contraception so they can enjoy sex without the worry of pregnancy.

I tried different forms of HC, one after the other, but a few months into each new regime I'd feel like I was losing my mind, with heavy, dark thoughts and a constantly clouded feeling.

Eighty per cent of women will, at some point, use HC. Not everyone has unwanted symptoms but, like many young women, for me the symptoms were preferable to the discomfort of having to share the responsibility and discuss safe sex with a partner.

Among the medical fraternity, this idea of switching off a female's cycle until she wants to conceive is accepted as a good idea. Ovulation just isn't considered that important. How do you think men would feel if we suggested that they suppress their testosterone cycle?

A recent Danish study with over one million participants supports the link between hormonal contraception and an increased risk of depression. It found that the relationship was most prevalent among teenage participants. Hormonal contraception was designed for adults, and the impact it has on brain development in young women is not well understood. More research is sorely needed.

What we do know is that of all the HC methods available, the only one that may allow regular ovulation and the production of your own hormones is the hormonal IUD — in Australia it's known as the Mirena. The copper IUD is also making a comeback because copper is toxic to sperm and non-hormonal.

I was almost twenty when I decided that I wanted my hormones back, and coming off the pill was like stepping out of a fog into a technicolour world.

Contraception is a very personal matter, and we all do the best we can with what we have. I know I paid a price, but I'm glad I didn't get pregnant as a teenager. If HC is as right as can be for you right now, then it's right. But, as always, keep checking in with how you feel. Keep listening to the messages your body is sending.

USE YOUR GIVE PHASE POWER

Look around you at everything that is wonderful about your life. Now, use your Give power to make it all even more wonderful. At work, in relationships, creatively . . . everything flowers at your touch. Yes, I did actually just write that as though I've been reading romance novels, but it's true! This week, you ARE a romance novel. The power of Do is a bit more of a blunt instrument whereas Give melts effortlessly into everyone and everything around you — greasing the wheels of your life, as it were.

Aim high, knowing that you have the energetic reserves and the confidence to pull it all off. You can afford to stay up a little later and know that if you burn the candle at both ends a bit now (within reason), you probably won't have to pay for it, so whatever it is that you're working on, give it your all. When the tap is running, let it flow. Progesterone also has a calming effect on our adrenal glands, so you are less likely to feel overwhelmed and stressed even if you have a lot going on (which you are liable to given this is the week of 'yes').

In the fog of your fabulousness, it's important to think back to your goals and dreams. Those seeds you sowed last week in your Do phase are now ripe for harvesting and so are you; don't leave them rotting on the vine. This is the time for the final push towards fabulous before you prepare for retreat.

It might feel frivolous to dedicate this week to self-celebration — to dancing in your gumboots and masturbating — and yes, there are more serious ways to harness this phase, but really, the best things are born from joy, and surely the world needs more of you at your most unbridled and joyous. Without being overly dramatic (what am I saying? I love being overly dramatic), WE'RE ALL GOING TO DIE ONE DAY AND WE DON'T KNOW WHEN. With this in mind, the least you can do is make the most of this moment, especially during this phase that so deserves to be made the most of. Here's how.

GIVE LOVE TO YOUR PASSION PROJECTS

With the influx of peaceful progesterone, your mojo swans in like she owns the place. Hopefully, after enough doing last week, you are able to dedicate some of this energy blast to your most treasured projects. Meet Shannah Mitchell, who says her best creative work is done here in Give:

> I'm a visual artist — a painter. Before tracking my cycle, I assumed that having good and bad painting days was just part of the process. What I then discovered was that these 'bad days' always fell roughly between Days 6 and 13 of my cycle [before she ovulated]. Over this time, I would avoid starting by doing washing, exercise and other odd jobs around the house. Sometimes I wouldn't even start at all. And when I did, I could never get into the headspace I needed to be in to make art. I would beat myself up every month for not doing what I thought I should be doing. Which would then have a

knock-on effect on my relationships with my family, and my home life. What I know now is that I can still work during this time [Do] because it's the only time of the month that I plan, make appointments, gather material and check over my equipment. I get so much done and I love it! The result is a huge increase in my productivity as it means I am in a better position at every other stage of the month to get out straight away and paint well. I am so grateful for this knowledge and knowing how to work and live more calmly and effectively.

Shannah's livelihood depends on her creativity (and really it isn't hard to argue that all of us depend on our creativity to some extent), and she recognises that if she uses the Do phase to set herself up for doing, she actually gets more creative work done in Give. Just another example of a rad lady going with her flow. There are no rules and we're all so different, but when you learn what to use each of *your* phases for, they all seem to flow more smoothly.

SHARE YOUR GENEROUS SPIRIT

If a problem shared is a problem halved, then surely when joy is shared it is doubled or tripled even. The biological backstory to this theory is that through our generosity at this time, we foster connections with those we love and rely on. In doing so, we prepare for a potential pregnancy, which will incur the need for a support system for our survival. *I have extra now, so I will share it with you because you need it, and then I get to benefit when you have extra and I need it.*

A woman in her post-ovulation phase who calls her menstruating friend to offer support is an excellent example of this perfect biological transaction. She has everything now, and the menstruator has sweet FA. Sometimes, I'll throw a message on one of my group chats saying, 'I have a full cup, who needs me? I can pick up your kids/wine or a rendang pie. Hit me up, I'm good for it all week.'

There are lots of ways to give. I find I cook more during my Give phase, or at least I enjoy cooking more when I do it. I like to 'whip up a cake' (not a phrase I normally even say out loud) and store it in a love heart tin. I get a real kick out of knowing it's there in the cupboard with icing on it, waiting to be dished out to whomever is lucky enough to cross my path. Sometimes the sweetest moments of connection are with complete strangers —, the wordless exchange of approval with other women in a fitting room, or forging an instant but fleeting bond over each other's life story in a toilet queue. Isn't life amazing?

We are hard-wired to share but never more so than now; you might find yourself literally giving someone the shirt off your back and then maybe strutting around shirtless in the sunlight (a fantasy scenario I'd like to see play out without resulting in arrest before I die). You will also be more inclined to see gifts or cards that would be just perfect for so-and-so during your Give phase, and research confirms that you are inclined to spend more money after ovulation (in your luteal phase) on gifts for loved ones and even more likely to donate to charity. This is known as 'prosociality' and was probably researched to determine when to advertise more efficiently to women. Some cycle-tracking apps took advantage of this by targeting women with different types of ads at different times of the month. Buyer beware indeed!

If you ordinarily find it hard to commit to purchases or treats for yourself, this is the time to do it. If you see some pink corduroy flares that you just have to have, yes you do. Have them. But if you're addicted to shopping, do yourself a favour and hide your credit card this week.

The takeaway here is to keep one foot on the ground, especially the next time you are accosted by charity workers who want you to save the whales/trees/planet — you are particularly prone to saying yes now and could be vulnerable to Commitment Without Consideration. But what do I know? Give to your heart's content. And as well as buying birthday presents, pre-write any cards needed over the coming weeks because next week you won't be feeling quite as emotionally generous, and writing cards while premenstrual can be onerous. Do it now, with a full heart.

CONNECT WITH OTHERS

I used to think that I was a completely spontaneous person and that I hated planning social engagements in advance because what if I got to the day and I didn't feel like doing the thing anymore? Now I know I'm a complete mistress to my body and that this is the week when I want to celebrate and connect — like clockwork. If I get too stuck in the Do phase and forget to make socialising a priority now, I can feel a bit forlorn if the Give phase comes around and I haven't got anything to look forward to and anyone to Give to. Make plans so that you don't miss out, and enjoy your summer fruits by sharing them. Plan a party or do something lovely for someone, just because. Fill your cup and everyone else's because next week you won't be quite so inclined to make the same kind of effort. Take your turn to host friends, and enjoy preparing a space that feels/smells/tastes/looks nice, or plan a picnic with a swim and a bushwalk. It doesn't need to be lavish or expensive, you yourself are quite enough.

If you have children, this is a lovely time to delight in them more than usual. Make extra time to hear about whatever slightly boring thing they are excited about, and go on adventures together doing exactly as they please at their chosen pace for some special family bonding.

If you have a partner, you are likely to feel more attracted to them now and want to express your desire and connection to them. As unsexy as it might sound, I plan for this and make an occasion out of being completely present for my partner so that he feels totally cherished, worshipped and supported. Later, when I retreat, he understands. Also, when I need to be cherished, I can rely on him to look after me, too. I didn't change my name when we got married but I routinely think about doing it in this phase.

Maybe you really like someone and you finally feel ready to tell them. Lucky them. If they don't reciprocate, your big egg energy means that you'll be best placed to handle it and more able to move on to the next exciting world of possibility. However, be forewarned that if you do go on a date, you will see the potential in a rock right now. *Mmm mmm . . . Stable, reliable, grounded, not bad.* Whoa, Nelly! Hold off on making long-term commitments while you are predisposed to seeing everyone as though the sun literally shines out of their ass.

I have more patience now and more energy to be supportive to others. This in action might mean helping someone with their workload, or offering a cup of tea (or wine) and a listening ear. You don't need to perform any grand gestures; a heart-to-heart with someone you've not seen in a while or with a friend who's been having a hard time could be all that is needed for them to feel supported and cared for. Make an effort to reach out and be there for your friends if you know that they need it, but also show them how much you appreciate them just because. Have you checked in recently and asked what is going on for them? It is so easy for us all to get caught up in ourselves and assume that people know they are loved. They might know it all right, but this is the time to really make them feel it. So go wave your magic love wand and share your gorgeous heart. Good friends are rare gems to be prized. The greatest gifts and the best balms to burnish a friendship are to really listen and to be truly present.

It isn't just good for our friends; it's good for us. Spending time with others, especially women, helps us to connect and feel stronger. It's like fuel, and the Give phase is the perfect time to give it and to get it.

If you are going through a time of isolation, this might be the week you notice a real yearning for close friends and connection. Now is a good time to reach out and cultivate new friendships when you're more likely to feel confident, outgoing and relaxed. Join a craft group, a dance class or a volunteer group, or just say hello to someone. If it doesn't go anywhere, what did you lose? Keep practising and never give up seeking out people who see you and feed your soul. Sometimes it takes a while to find your people, but they are out there and this is a good time to look for them.

HAVE DIFFICULT CONVERSATIONS AND PROBLEM-SOLVE

You have a super-optimistic lens right now. Everything is about 32 per cent rosier than usual, so use this time to navigate your own big hurdles and also to support your friends and the people closest to you.

While we're at it, here's some real talk: it's time to sing 'Kumbaya', to dig deep and deal with whatever proverbial stone has been stuck in your shoe. If there is something big (or even small) between you and someone you care about, or something at home or work that's been weighing on your mind, address it now. You have a greater capacity for empathy and diplomacy, so gird your loins and use your smooth-talking ability to do some emotional/social maintenance.

Prepare your thoughts and schedule some time with whoever it is. It isn't always easy to do this just because you're high on pro-gesterone but this is when it IS easiest, and every time you practise deep connection and communication, you build your relationship muscles and get better at dealing with conflict in a positive way. Maybe there was a misunderstanding or maybe the other person is completely oblivious; whatever the cause or the reason, talking from a place of openness and kindness never hurts.

Am I overreacting? Is it just me? Issues are always bigger and uglier when they are trapped in our minds. Questions like these can go round and round and sap precious energy, so shake it out and burst the bubble. Take away its power and show someone how much faith you have in your friendship by being brave enough to call out 'the thing'.

Now is also the perfect time to rectify any friendly fire that may have been flung (in Take, or even Do), and to revisit the issue with a fresh heart. If the result of the coming-together session is hearing some painful truths, this will be the easiest time to hear them. None of us is perfect and it isn't easy to hear that you hurt someone or messed up, but in your Give phase your ego is best placed to take on some constructive criticism. After all, this is how we grow.

Wash, rinse, repeat.

PLAY TO YOUR STRENGTHS AT WORK

Your powers of persuasion are at an all-time high this week, so if you want to change something in order to improve your life or someone else's, this is the time to best use your bargaining power. Negotiate away. What do you need? From your parents? A partner? At work? From your local MP? Write down what you really want and, if you can, plan to have these important, high-stakes conversations this week so that you can benefit from your peak confidence and give yourself the best chance of getting what you need. You won't always get it, but you might.

Lead the charge for change with an ability to connect. Your capacity for empathy and compassion is one of the hallmarks of the Give phase. Look at how the Prime Minister of New Zealand Jacinda Ardern has used this to run an entire country. In an

interview with BBC News, she said, 'I'm very proudly an empa-
thetic, compassionately driven politician. We teach kindness
and empathy and compassion to our children, but then we
somehow when it comes to political leadership, want a complete
absence of that. So I am trying to chart a different path.' So can
you. Follow your heart and others will, too.

SEEK OUT COLLABORATORS AND GROW YOUR NETWORK

I encourage you to consider the ramifications for your 'non-baby'
pregnancy and ask yourself which big dream is begging to be
born? And WHO will help you birth it? Who will support you to
raise the thing? We live in such a culture of individualism, a
culture where independence is prized and where we feel powerful when we don't rely on anybody. You know what? That's bullshit. Great things are burgeoned by telling your friends
and colleagues your most excellent ideas and getting help
when it's needed.

When you sat with your seeds during Dream and Do and
teased out all of the smaller tasks that needed ticking off in order
for your dream goal to be realised, you might have noted that
you possibly aren't the best woman to tackle all of them. That's
why you get help. No woman is an island, and no woman is better
placed to ask for help (or for anything at all, really) than you are
right now. So think carefully about who you can reach out to, and
how. The power of your reach is prolific, so don't commit unless
you are sure, but once you are, lock it down.

If you get a fabulous idea that involves someone else and a wild proposition that is equal parts exciting and overwhelming, sit on it for at least an hour before you press send. If you still feel excited, what the hell, go for it.

Your enthusiasm is infectious now, so of course people will want to be a part of whatever exciting plan you are working on. Reach out now, not just to potential collaborators (old and new), but also to potential mentors for support and encouragement to help grow your projects. Build your network into a brains/womb trust that you can turn to for advice and support. Remember that you are an important part of other people's networks, too. This is how men have done so well in the past — by looking out for each other. There's a lot of truth in the phrase 'It isn't what you know, but who you know', so get knowing.

It could be as simple as saying, 'Hey, I have this great idea. It's [fill in your great idea here] and I'm wondering if you could offer your advice/give me an idea about/would like to chat about collaborating with me?' If it's a major idea, put together a one-page pitch so they can see that you are serious and that they should be, too. Chances are they'll be thrilled to have been asked and have a chance to share their goodness with you.

As you approach the end of the Give phase, ask yourself if you've sufficiently tapped the universe to give enough love to whatever is important to you. Have you given your dreams enough of an opportunity for them to thrive? Goodness and support is out there, you just need to ask for it. Sometimes you need to give it to get it. Get the ball rolling now while you still have the gift of the gab, and next month you can follow up again if you want to. Give it a go!

CHALLENGES IN THE GIVE PHASE

Even the sweet spot of the cycle can have some bones in it. While this phase might seem like the easiest one, every light has its shadow. Whatever cycle we're working with, healthy boundaries can help us all to take care of ourselves and manage better.

NOT GIVING IT ALL AWAY

When you feel like you have the world on a string and more to give than 'Daddy' Warbucks, it can be a pretty exhilarating feeling to just give and give as though there is no tomorrow. But there is a tomorrow and one or two or three after that, and then before you know it, you'll be in the Take phase and your future self will not appreciate you having given away every last available shred. What are you giving your time, love and energy to? How do you catch yourself from losing balance?

Here's one very practical piece of advice: do not leave your Give self in charge of your diary for any extended period of time. She'll promise the rest of your week, month and who knows what else away. Your capacity for generosity now really is at peak levels, but you need to be aware of the boundaries of this bounty. You are prone to extreme acts of passion, so do not commit to big-ticket items that would do well to be run through a whole cycle. For example, don't volunteer for any enormous projects, offer to donate a kidney or try to sort out the major messes in other people's lives without asking, 'Can I think about it?' You might feel like Mother Teresa this week, but next week will be different. And don't, whatever you do, scroll through the pet adoption pages without an emotional spotter on stand-by to help you resist seven of their cute little orphaned faces. I have a friend who bought a tiny puppy on the spur of the moment while in her Give phase. Her miniature pinscher, Mochi, was illegally cute and about 20 centimetres long.

Unfortunately, Mochi also turned out to be an acute sufferer of 'small dog syndrome', and was quite aggressive towards her child and existing dog, a great Dane. And by the time she arrived in her Take phase, Gigi lamented, 'I made a mistake!' But she swore she would see out another month in order for this decision to run through a full cycle. Months after the 'longest ever adjustment', Mochi has mellowed out and everyone's happy, but the moral of this story is to check before you commit.

Are you saying yes because you genuinely want to or because you feel you should? Leave some rubber room in your schedule so that you can say yes to things spontaneously as they happen and don't feel overloaded or too pressured. You might feel responsible for every stray animal/person/half-finished work project, but you are not a social worker — unless you are, but even then remember not to spend too much of yourself in this phase or next week you'll be cursing yourself and everyone else.

SETTING LIMITS WITH SOCIAL MEDIA

During this phase, you might feel more driven to share your fabulousness online. And why not share a banging selfie? After all, this is a time to celebrate, and feeling good about yourself is definitely something worth celebrating. Just make sure you don't become reliant on other people validating you to feel that you are worth it. Share the selfie or don't, but either way, know deeply that you are worth celebrating.

The other thing to watch out for here is frittering away your Give powers online. Certainly, I have sent a few DMs during that phase filled with excitement and a collaboration suggestion that has evolved into a real-life situation. But if you spend your giving virtually at the expense of giving in real life, you'll be denying your deep human need for real and meaningful connection and purpose. This can lead to disappointment that might come to the boil in the Take phase, too.

Be open to creating situations that give your light a real opportunity to shine and be reflected back to you. Share it with deserving subjects, and enjoy seeing your gifts manifested as love and kindness in others. Remember that this power is not something to be concentrated into an electronic device and diluted into an imaginary ether. You need to look it in the face and drink it up.

NOT FEELING LIKE GIVING AT ALL (AKA WHERE IS MY JOY?)

If you come to this phase feeling like you didn't get enough time to properly 'do' last week or have a chance to answer the call or the quest that was rightfully yours, you won't feel quite as ready to party on the mountaintops of Peak Fabulous, let alone host a party for anyone else. Did you back yourself in the Do phase or did you hamstring your mojo? If you didn't use your Do power for its intended purpose, you can feel a bit devastated in Give, and FOMO can give way to AMO (Actually Missing Out). It's quite okay to feel disappointed in whatever phase you are in, but if you feel it now, ask yourself what it is you might have missed last week in your Do phase and then make a note to focus on it next time.

If you feel terrible or just off during this phase, it could be a sign of a hormonal imbalance. In the same way that we can be sensitive to coffee and foods in a unique way, some people reel at the elevated hormones and suffer emotionally because of them. There are lots of ways you can learn to support your hormonal health naturally, and if you need help or more knowledge, I encourage you to seek it out.

If you are abnormally stressed, it's possible that you won't ovulate and get to enjoy the benefits of progesterone at all. It isn't normal to be so stressed that you don't ovulate, but it is common to have anovulatory cycles sometimes. Think about it: if you are under heaps of stress and producing a lot of stress hormones, your body makes the call that this isn't going to be an ideal environment to conceive in. If your stress is such that you aren't ovulating, it's probably having other effects, too, so see this as a sign to get help.

Re-read the section on Giving to yourself (page 180) and remember that you are a divine creature, perfect the way you are and created to feel joy. In short, if you don't feel like being generous with others, perhaps you could be more generous with your dear self.

NOT WANTING TO MOVE ON TO TAKE

If you felt like maybe last week was the real you, then this week you are sure about it. 'No, really,' you say as you toss your hair over your shoulder and catch your reflection in the nearest shiny surface, 'this is definitely the real me!' What can commonly happen in this part of the cycle is that we feel so fantastic that we take it for granted that this is who we really are — someone with constant energy and time for others, someone who wakes up feeling generous and enjoys being able to continuously give.

And after riding the high of those good feelings, coming to the end of this phase can be like paying a huge bill after a fantastic dinner with cocktails and dessert: *How much?* It can feel disappointing, like everything was going so well and then the rug just got pulled from under you and now you feel so scratchy and cranky. 'What is *wrong* with me?' you wail. 'Last week everything was so great; why do I want to bite things?'

Be gentle with these feelings as you transition to the next phase. Let them remind you to stay soft to change.

Notice what you love about the Give phase and learn how to best use it. Feel satisfied that you gave your best and that those around you got a good dose of your giving self. It *was* enough, and it will be again in due course.

PREPARiNG TO TAKE

The Give part of the cycle has become the poster girl for the 'ideal female': generous, helpful, servile, happy, accepting, nurturing, kind, maternal . . . But can you imagine how it would be to be like this every single day? When you period like a queen you enjoy the depths of each phase, and when it's time to let go, you take a deep breath and welcome the next part of yourself. You let it in and pull up a chair.

After a few days of progesterone-fuelled bliss, take a moment to check in with yourself. Phew! This week can be a heady ride, but now you know what's coming — you know where this train is headed. Next stop is the Take phase via PMS station, so make life easy for yourself: DON'T PUT IMPORTANT THINGS OFF HERE.

Trust me, whether you've got a big deadline, a difficult email to write or a tough project to handle at work, you will NOT want to deal with it next week. Leaving things to the last minute only puts you under pressure and means you arrive at the cave's entrance ready to flop, only to be forced to drag yourself a little bit farther while you finish off whatever task you've been putting off.

TOP UP YOUR TANK BEFORE THE GATE CLOSES

The end of this phase is a blurry line. Sometimes it's a fade-out, sometimes it comes with a bang. Your transition day is the day you cross over from feeling a joyous ease and a connection to all things wonderful to a kind of crunchy feeling accompanied by a not-so-joyous shorter fuse and increased likelihood of feeling snappy.

If you gave away every ounce you had during your Give phase and you've skidded into your Take phase at about Day 21, unprepared and energetically on empty, some big feelings might knock you sideways. The wheels can fall off the whole operation, and you can feel prickly as hell. The Take phase is immeasurably harder (for you and others in close proximity) when you feel like you have nothing left. Ease this transition by milking the last of your Give phase and donating the proceeds back to yourself. A worthy cause indeed.

Remember to breathe (like really breathe). You take around 20,000 breaths every day so make at least a few of them like special treats. Think about how you can create a ritual for yourself to let go of your Give phase and welcome your Take phase. It's going to last a week, or maybe even longer, and your cup is about to empty, so top it up as soon as you know that your Give gate is closing. If you start to slow down and do this, you might not even notice much of a transition at all.

This ritual might involve doing some yoga to move any crunchy feelings through your body before they get a chance to take root. It might involve meditation; set yourself up to be in a good frame of mind, and use incense or oils such as lavender or a candle to create a calm, lovely space. Go somewhere quiet and comfortable, and use an app or an online meditation video to help to soothe your body and mind. Set an intention. This could be really simple, something like *I am patient with myself,* or *I am present.* It could be forgiving yourself if you don't do something perfectly or just slowing down while you brush your teeth. Never forget, your body is doing a lot on the inside. Be nice to it, and stay soft and open to welcome your Take phase. And now?

Batten down the hatches, bitches. Your most magical self is just around the corner, and she has big business to handle.

Day 18 Dream Journal

I dreamed that I was floating down a river, stretched out on my back and smiling like Baloo from *The Jungle Book.* Lying on my chest was a dear friend, taking refuge as we floated along.

CHAPTER 7

TAKE

Imagine a queen who's just thrown a huge, fantastic party that lasted for days. It was a wonderful time for one and all but now she's feeling a bit frazzled. She has nothing to wear and no clean knickers left. There are wine rings all over the benches. And the toilet? Ergh. Why are people so . . . peopley? She yearns for time alone to do whatever she wants. She takes a deep breath and one last look before she shuts the door and turns away from, well, everything really. She begins her descent down the mountain in exactly the fashion that feels good to her. She gathers her wits and starts walking, swinging her arms and punching away the dragons. There is a journey ahead but she knows this is her time to take before she does it all over again.

When you're ovulating you're all, 'Yes! Thank you! Hi there! Hello, thanks for coming! So lovely to see you!' You reach the zenith of your biggest and brightest self. If the Give phase was all about being with your friends and family, and bathing them in your brilliance as your cup runneth over, Take is all about prioritising and being with yourself while that same cup empties fast. It can still be brilliant, just a different kind of brilliant.

This magic is not so much for sharing; it's more about protection and distillation. Once your hormones start to decline, your whole being aches in protest, particularly at the loss of progesterone. After the intense loveliness of the Give phase, where everything seemed at least 39 per cent more wonderful, now life can suddenly feel about 92 per cent more vexing.

This can certainly be a challenging time. After all, you're coming to the end of your cycle and preparing to let go again. Take is the last lap of the race, and it's the most tiring and demanding one. Hence the need to run it at your own pace and also to retreat and scaffold, which I'll explain throughout this chapter.

Just as we need to coax out our Dream phase power, Take requires a little seduction, too. There are ways to take care of yourself, not only to avoid fallout, but also to help you use this phase for good. This is your time to Take: take the biggest piece of cake, take the easy way out, and most of all, take time to be creative during what is possibly the most potent phase. Do prepared you to Give, and now Take will prepare you to Dream.

The ocean does not apologise for its depth and the mountains do not seek forgiveness for the space they take and so, neither shall I. — *Becca Lee (writer and poet)*

KNOW YOUR

take PHASE

FROM DAY 21ISH UNTIL DAY 28ISH
(THE DAY BEFORE YOU BLEED)

WHY IS IT HAPPENING?

Your egg came and went, and soon
so will the 'nest'. Your hormones
plummet to prepare you to start again.

YOGA POSE:
SEATED SPINAL
TWIST

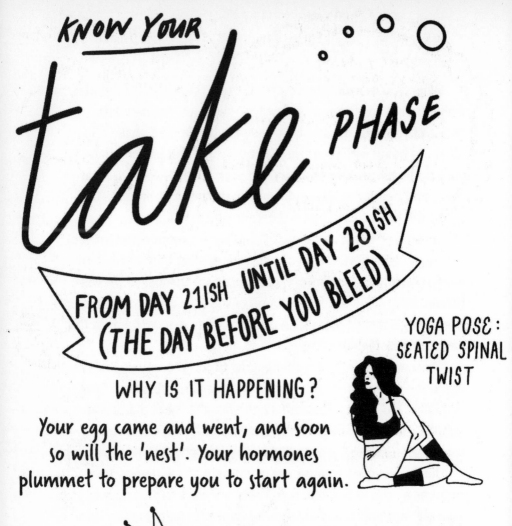

your superpower is...

To take stock,
to see everything in
sharp focus, to take
no crap.

DO NOT DISTURB

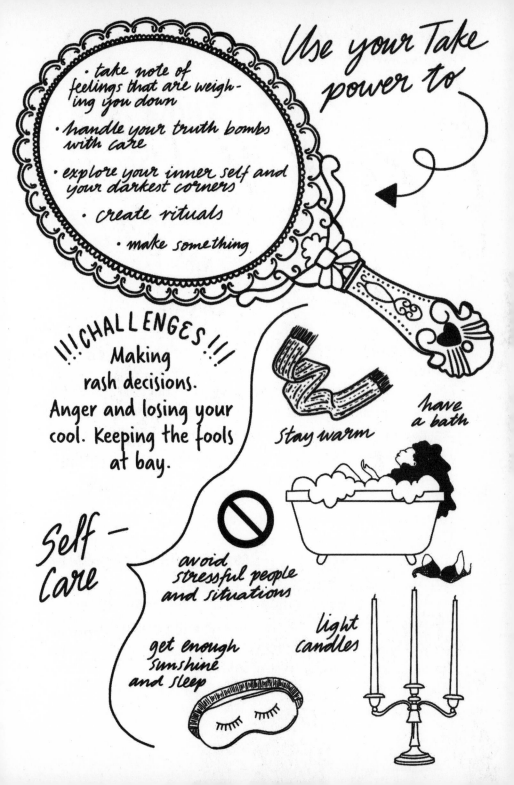

Use your Take power to

- take note of feelings that are weighing you down
- handle your truth bombs with care
- explore your inner self and your darkest corners
- create rituals
- make something

!!!CHALLENGES!!!
Making rash decisions. Anger and losing your cool. Keeping the fools at bay.

Self-Care

stay warm

have a bath

avoid stressful people and situations

get enough sunshine and sleep

light candles

GET TO KNOW YOUR TAKE PHASE

I often realise I've moved into the Take phase when I hurt myself. I bang my hip on the kitchen bench or I stub my toe. Possibly, I incur these injuries more frequently when entering the kitchen at speed because I'm so starving, I need to snack at the fridge. Give yourself a rub and S L O W down; it's time to take it easier.

Remember, there are high levels of inflammatory proteins called prostaglandins circulating in your bloodstream right now. They are necessary — eventually causing the breakdown of your endometrial lining so you'll have a period — but they also affect the rest of your body. This is why you can feel a bit loose in the tummy and maybe even like you have a mild head cold.

The increased sensitivity associated with this phase also means that your pain threshold is lower and your senses are more liable to feel overloaded. Lights are too bright, and everything sounds louder. The sound of an exhaust fan left on or cutlery clanking in the sink is enough to cause me genuine brain damage (even if someone else is doing the dishes). My skin feels prickly, particularly during the final throes (the night before my period comes). I can't get to sleep, I can't get comfortable and I wish I could crawl out of my whole body and go to Vanuatu.

You're also more likely to get sick now because your immune system is at its weakest, so it's important to take better care of yourself than usual, both physically and emotionally — it's all connected. Anything you do now to look after your mental health is a worthwhile investment. Start employing some of the self-care ideas from the Dream phase now, and consider this as preventative medicine as you move closer to your period.

As with each of the phases, your experience will be unique to you. But common to all of us is that during this much-maligned time of the month, women bear the brunt of societal misunderstanding. There is almost as much stigma around PMS as there is around periods.

No wonder we grit our teeth, push through this week and feel relieved once it's over. If we do have any big feelings, they are discounted with the classic: 'Oh, you're just premenstrual'. This handy catch-all has served to keep women quiet, to remind us that we're not allowed to get furious. Never mind that sometimes shit is f%cked and maybe after putting up with it all month long now you've finally had enough.

That's normally where the PMS story ends. People tell us we're being unreasonable, we expect to feel crappy, we do feel crappy and a begrudging tolerance sets in. It hides out in our wombs, in our tight shoulders, in our shallow breaths and clenched fists, and it settles between our eyes. It gets in the fecking way.

So where's the superpower hiding in this turd sandwich?

What if there was a better way? What if we could channel this phase into a superpower just like we do in the other three phases? And what if this superpower just happened to be the most bad-assiest of them all?

Good news, friend: it is.

PREMENSTRUAL? AVOID THESE THINGS

There are many activities you can and should do in this amazing and powerful phase, and we'll get to those in a moment. But there are also some things you should definitely *not do* on the spur of the moment, and these include:

💜 Indulging in a big night without drinking plenty of water. There are times in the month that you can get away with indulgence at little expense; this week is not one of them.

💜 Booking in for hair-removal procedures that involve extraction. Schedule these torture sessions for after your period during the Do or Give phases (or never).

💜 Drinking coffee if you are sensitive to caffeine during this phase, unless you're prepared to have a tight jaw all week.

💜 Getting a pixie cut or walking around with scissors for too long. My friend Tarryn says, 'Sometimes I want to symboli-cally cut all my hair off, give the middle finger to the patriar-chy and free myself of its constraints. But baldness isn't the answer, true power comes from within.'

💜 Breaking up with him/her unless you know for sure and this isn't the first time you've felt this way. (If it is the first time but you are certain, use the courage of this phase to push you on — with the blessing of everyone reading this book.)

♥ Buying a one-way ticket to Vegas. Is this ever a good idea?

♥ Exposing yourself to things you know will depress you.

I actually checked my period tracker to work out if I could handle my first listen of Nick Cave's new album. Turns out I'll be ready in two weeks. — Abbe May (singer–songwriter and human rights campaigner)

Day 31 Dream Journal

I dreamed I was dancing naked — whirling like a dervish, and I woke up feeling less tight and more free.

HONOUR THE TRANSITION INTO TAKE

💜 Wear something dark and witchy.

💜 Put on dramatic lipstick and a smoky eye, or whatever expresses the state of your current inner self.

💜 Light a candle and some incense.

💜 Play some sad-girl music and enjoy the melancholy.

💜 Play mad-girl music and dance it out.

💜 Move your hips to get connected to your centre — back and forth, in circles, whatever feels good.

💜 Sing along loudly and/or cry if you want to.

💜 Make time to play or make a mess. Retreat to a creative space or set up a 'making station' somewhere you can leave your things out, all set up, so you can come back to them throughout this phase whenever the making mood strikes.

💜 Tune in to whatever your body is aching for, and then give it to yourself freely.

💜 Give yourself a foot massage.

💜 Use self-pleasure to manage stress or anxiety.

💜 Have a bath with bath salts if you feel achy.

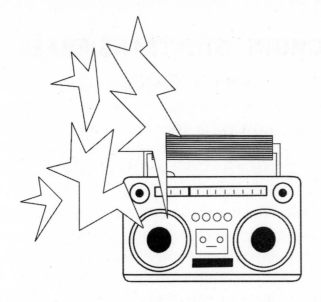

TAKE PHASE ESSENTIALS

♥ Art supplies and a journal

♥ A playlist to dance and maybe cry to

♥ Essential oils to mix with a nice carrier oil (almond oil, perhaps) for self-massage, or to add to the bath or a foot spa (a bucket will do). A few drops of oil in a homemade spritzer is nice, too. Jasmine is good for cramps and feeling sensual; neroli is uplifting and relaxing; and rose is nice when you are feeling low or sad.

♥ A digital thermometer to predict your period due date

♥ Treats, but especially dark chocolate

TRACKING YOUR TAKE PHASE

The Take phase begins as the Give glow starts to wear thin. For example, in a 31-day cycle I would ovulate by around Day 17/18 and move into Take around Day 24/25. If I ovulated at Day 15, my cycle would be shorter and I'd know to look out for the transition sooner. However, it can be difficult to pinpoint *exactly* when the Take phase begins because there are no definitive signs. One minute you're enjoying the boost in your cup size and the next, just going over a speed bump is enough to cause you genuine breast pain.

Take can sneak up on you, especially if you've been a bit lax with tracking during the Give phase. This is common because everything seems effortless and wonderful and *la, la, la. Life is great and I'm so busy living it that it hardly warrants a mention!* Until of course it isn't. But if you stick with the tracking — monitoring how you feel on various days and phases of your cycle — as you approach this final stage, you'll be able to finetune your responses and transition into Take more comfortably.

Even if your cycle is a bit all over the place, it's good to get into the habit of reflecting and listening to what your body and your heart need. Pay attention to the way you feel physically *and* emotionally, and note any changes commonly associated with this time, such as tiredness, depression, irritability, headaches, muscle aches, breast tenderness, bloating, increased appetite and skin outbreaks.

Almost everyone with a cycle will notice some of these changes around this week — they are symptoms of what is known as premenstrual syndrome, or PMS. The word 'syndrome' takes something that is very normal and common to the female experience, and pathologises it. The word implies that there is something medically wrong with us at this time of the month by using a term often associated with disease. And dis-*ease* may certainly be felt if it seems that most of society doesn't respect or understand this time of the month. But how different could your experience of this time be if you were well supported?

Occasionally, I hardly notice the transition from Give to Take at all, but this is no accident; it's because when I know Take is coming, I'm able to shift my focus and prepare. My premenstrual complaints are negligible, but it doesn't always work out that way.

By tracking and collecting information on yourself, you'll know what to expect and be able to support yourself accordingly. Not only will you have fewer surprise PMS attacks, but the symptoms will give way to a new set of traits to be recorded: a deeper sense of connection to yourself and profound moments of strength, clarity, inspiration and creativity. You can plan for how you want to use this superpower, too.

UNLOCKING YOUR SUPERPOWER

While you may mourn the passing of the summer of your Give phase, you'll still get the occasional warm day in the autumn of your cycle, and there is much creative energy to be harnessed if you know how to make the most of it. Autumn is my favourite season because it feels like a beginning. The heat fades and the earth exhales and the real work begins. According to the Indigenous Noongar calendar, in Western Australia autumn is

Djeran season, with cool nights and dewy mornings. It's the time of red flowers, and this means preparing your shelter for the season ahead.

It's true that your biggest, most heinous feelings can crop up now. And I'm talking venomous, deepest, darkest rage and vitriolic teeth-clenching, nostril-flaring angst. Feeling jealous, cranky, short-fused; basically, any big horrific feeling you can imagine is more likely to burn in on a Harley Davidson and tear down your emotional street doing wheelies and burnouts. If you are early in your menstruating career, these feelings can be alarming and cause you genuine suffering. Remember to breathe and to give them some room — really breathe. Sometimes, like a canary in the coalmine, heinous feelings are powerful indicators that shouldn't be ignored. Other times they surface because of an emotional backlog that we only notice once we're without the hormonal buffers of the previous weeks. A bit of column A, bit of column B — it can be hard to tell in the heat of the moment.

The good news is that you can channel these big feelings and use them to face the darkest parts of yourself with grace and courage; to sift through the rubble for the rubies in the dust. These gems are your greatest treasures, and the challenges within them are your biggest teachers. The more you understand this part of you, the better you become at facing any challenge. It's how we practise our power, and it's good practise for life.

Suppress what you feel in this phase and you'll miss out on the gold because putting a lid on the harder emotions also puts a big lid on the positive aspects of this phase. I didn't always love this phase, but now that I do, it's where I reap the greatest rewards. It's when I feel the fiercest. The power lies in channelling your feelings.

In this last phase, you can either come down off the mountain the easy way or the hard way. I'm sure you know about the hard way, so let's talk about how to scaffold with self-care. This will not only help you this week, but it will also help in your upcoming Dream phase. Think of it as building a shelter for winter, as in the Djeran season.

FEED YOURSELF LIKE YOU ARE YOUR OWN CHILD

There is no hunger like the hunger of a premenstrual woman. I have a friend with whom I share a not-so-secret love of 'hand-bag chicken' (the hot roasted kind from a supermarket). And at this time in our cycles, we find it is best enjoyed, as the name suggests, from the bag, with our bare hands. This is not a time to deny yourself — your skyrocketing metabolism simply demands more food than you needed last week. Your body is working hard already to process the high levels of hormones that came with ovulation, and you can help by getting enough fibre from vegetables and drinking water. Junk food will only add to the load (and worsen the PMS symptoms).

If you need more support with alleviating symptoms, consult your practitioner about taking daily supplements of magnesium and vitamin B6, as well as filling your own dark-chocolate prescription (you're welcome).

Eat. Eat until you are satisfied. Tear the meat from the bones, suck the marrow and lick your fingers like the premenstrual wild woman you are.

EXERCISE

With your body on stand-by for a potential pregnancy, your energy is fading. Don't be disappointed if you aren't able to exercise as hard or for as long as you normally do. If you need a rest day (or days), take it. Your body is prioritising, so do whatever exercise you like but consider lessening the intensity.

If you are feeling overwhelmed with the world around you (or inside you), moving your body will help burn some of this fizzy energy and elevate your mood with endorphins. A walk or even just a few salutes to the sun will soften your body and make it easier for you to relax deeply when the time to Dream comes.

There are lots of good ways to exercise and feel more connected to yourself, and this is important as you get closer to the void of PMS. Try non-contact boxing or lifting weights to help you feel grounded and strong. Yoga, Pilates or tai chi will help to balance and centre you, or dance to feel creative.

In July 2019, the American women's soccer team won the World Cup. They credited a secret weapon that gave them an edge. It was (drum roll, please) cycle tracking! Each player's training schedule was bespoke to her cycle, working in sync with her body and telling her when to work harder for more gain, when to get more sleep, what to eat at what time of the month and so on. One journalist wrote that Rose Lavelle scored the game-winning goal 'in spite of being premenstrual' and got her period the next day. *In spite of?* Google her goal and watch it. You'll see it is pure power. Rose channelled every shred of power she had and scored this goal not *in spite of* being premenstrual but BECAUSE SHE WAS. She used it. So can you.

LET GO OF DO AND GIVE

First things first: take a deep breath and reflect on the last two weeks. You've just come off the back of two pretty massive phases: Do (pre-ovulation) and Give (post-ovulation), where you absolutely peaked in terms of the resources you had available. You've basically climbed the two biggest mountains of your month and it felt so good; no wonder it's a hard part of yourself to say goodbye to. Do and Give always get all the glory, and I reckon this gives your Take self the absolute shits.

Hence the pressure we feel, internally and externally, to maintain unrealistic levels of productivity and generosity. And here's the rub: if you feel the need to be all things to all people and you expect yourself to maintain the emotional and physical expenditure of the last two weeks when you are actually on your way to empty, of course everything will feel harder. *Of course* you'll feel irritable/snap/cry/explode.

You are about to tear down some internal walls (physical and emotional) but no one knows or sees this work, which, it bears repeating, is HOW WE ALL EXIST. We're expected to carry on as usual. No one talks about who we are for around 25 per cent of our fertile lives. If 'usual' means being the emotional and practical logisticator (and yes, I know that isn't a real word, but I'm premenstrual; don't come at me) of your family/friend group/workspace, or if you are the person who keeps mental tabs on the contents of the fridge/washing pile/lost-sock drawer/homework tally, then prickly feelings will peak in prickliness now.

SET PROTECTIVE BOUNDARIES

Pre-empt the pricks and gently let people know that you'll be taking a back seat for a while, and assure them that everyone will be happier this way. Thank them in advance and say you appreciate their support. If you don't feel supported to delegate, remember, *you* are your greatest ally. Support yourself as best you can and know that you will feel less crappy if you feed your soul. If you don't laugh, you cry. And if you don't cry, you scream. But hey, why don't you smile more? It's enough to make you growl.

If you deny the realities of your emotional bank balance and keep spending yourself (particularly on other people) when you just don't have anything left, then the debt can be crippling and the fallout monumental. The end result is having to allocate even more energy later to the emotional clean-up, putting you further in debt as you head for a more difficult period in the Dream phase.

To that end, here are five take-care-of-yourself tactics to put into action this week.

1. **Channel your limited resources to yourself**
   Feeling that you have nothing to give to those around you can be hard, and it takes real resolve to mind yourself here. Assure yourself that you gave enough already, and that you will have time and energy for others soon. Right now, you need to channel this power in the best way that you can.

2. **Be smart about who you spend time with**
   Apart from the absolute essentials (work, school, appointments), don't expect as much from yourself in the couple of

days before you bleed. Set some boundaries about who you will and won't spend time with. Schedule necessary interactions with any emotional vampires during Do and Give (or never). Some people will defend their right to be miserable until the death and then blame you for it. Avoid them, especially now. You can't afford them.

3. Relieve pressure

If you crave time alone without pressure, fast-track high-priority tasks, such as finishing most of a project/job that can't wait until your first few days of bleeding are over. Save whatever time is left for yourself, to spend alone.

4. Be okay with being brief

Just because you are less inclined to punctuate your communication with carefully considered emojis doesn't mean you are some kind of monster; it means you are only giving what you have available.

5. Disconnect, if you can

Turn off your phone for a while. You are coming down the mountain, preparing to enter the temple of yourself at menstruation, so take time to make yourself spiritually presentable and cull the crap. Period coach Claire Baker (yes, that's a thing!) recommends deleting all of your addictive apps just for a while. Great advice.

FORGET FOMO AND EMBRACE JOMO

Ever gone out because you felt you should? 'Yes,' said everyone ever. You've probably had times where even though you really *wanted* to want to go out, the reality was that you would have been better off at home.

The fear of missing out can be a powerful motivator. *I'm no quitter*, you say to yourself, determined not to let anyone down and to enjoy the commitment you wish you hadn't made. You *must* do what you said you'd do, dammit! Even though you are devastated because your best jeans aren't fully dry yet and the hair dryer isn't helping. You couldn't find the right earrings and you couldn't get your eyeliner angle to be the same on both eyes, *DAMMIT*. You arrive at the venue late, the music is exactly the type that you least want to be hearing, and your friends aren't where they said they'd be. You yawn through your nostrils and suddenly your inner voice shouts, *What am I doing here?!*

Good question. I don't actually know, you think to yourself. You ponder the alternative activities you could have participated in tonight, things like:

- Having a two-hour bath with a book and snacks
- Going to a movie by yourself (in dark glasses and a blankie)
- Sitting in a café (alone), facing the wall and ordering a hot chocolate with extra chocolate or extra everything because you are ravenous on account of your hyper-metabolic state

💜 Literally anything else, such as eating cardboard but mostly the delicious alternative of ...

💜 Doing nothing

Even if you're a wild extrovert, everyone needs time alone. And when you're getting ready to meet your most precious self at menstruation, you are least likely to regret choosing to be alone rather than spending time with people that you don't 100 per cent want to be with. You don't need that kind of distraction. Forget FOMO. Luxuriate in the joy of missing out instead and never look back.

USiNG YOUR TAKE PHASE POWER

Now that you know how to call forth your Take power, how will you use it? What magic will you conjure? What will you turn your majesty to? How will you cloak yourself in magnificence?

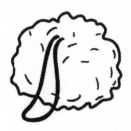

USE YOUR POO-COLOURED GLASSES

Consider what it actually means to be premenstrual: after using all of your lovely ovulatory energy on family and friends, expressing your gorgeous self in all of the ways that you do and perfecting that luscious nest deep inside you, your body has just cottoned on that you will not be making a baby this month. As a result, you lose those hormonal buffers and everything starts to come into super-sharp focus.

Forget the rose-tinted glasses you were wearing in the last phase. Now you're looking at the world through a new lens, and it's slightly poo-tinted. Things that might ordinarily escape your attention are now glaringly obvious. It's as if your eyes and your intuition were trained to sniff out crap. In fact, it's as though you have a *calling* to seek and call out crap. You can't stand injustice, and your inner self goes in to bat for you like a bloody cheerleader.

This is natural and good because you *need* to call out crap that is crap, and you need to let things go. If you wore those rosy glasses all month, you'd hold on to every toxic friend for dear life, as well as every drawing you'd done since you were six, and NOBODY HAS TIME FOR THAT, or space. Especially now, dear reader.

To take advantage of those heightened crap detectors, you must channel your focus. Otherwise the glare will burn holes in unsuspecting victims (including you).

Do *not* use this super-critical focus to analyse any of the following things:

💜 **Anything at all about your face, hair or body.** Please leave your skin/thighs/ankles/earlobes/nose alone (see self-care tips on page 209). If you must pop something gargantuan, do it once with clean hands. Being gentle with yourself is paramount, with your thoughts, your heart and your skin.

💜 **Cryptic text messages.** Sure, you could read that message in three different ways, but before you go too deep, put the phone down and consider dialling up the sunshine just a notch or two. Make sure you aren't training your crap focus on how you feel others see you. This applies to digesting texts, emails, facial expressions or any form of communication from others. Breathe. Assume that the person sending the information did it with the best intentions.

💜 **The state of the world.** Ugh. During this phase, the state of the government and/or the environment can cause you genuine grief. There are many injustices being committed right in front of our eyes, and we do need to address them in order to make sense of what's going on and figure out how we can personally respond. This can be a good time to do that (see Channel the fury on page 228), but don't spend too long here or you might find that you feel swamped and paralysed by fury or grief.

Write your feelings down, talk to someone, or make a note to come back to this issue in your Dream phase and mull over it then. When you get to Do, you can act on it. Right now, you can do something small and still significant, but be mindful of what you consume digitally and socially — be protective of your headspace.

🖤 **Yourself.** A little bit of self-doubt is okay and can help keep our egos in check, but don't give it a megaphone and start taking notes. Instead, give it lasagne and see if you feel better.

CHANNEL THE FURY

Sometimes, anger — specifically the anger that pops up in this week of your cycle — can be used productively.

Meet Gabby Edlin, founder and CEO of a UK charity called Bloody Good Period, set up in response to the needs of refugee women and asylum seekers during their periods. What started as a whip-around on Facebook grew into an enterprise that now supplies 40 asylum-seeker drop-in centres in London and Leeds with menstrual products, because everybody has the right to a bloody good period. Indeed.

When I asked Gabby how she uses her cycle, she was quick with her answers:

🖤 She takes it easier during her period and encourages all of the 'bleeders' who work for her to do the same.

🖤 She goes hard in her Do phase to make as much progress as she can for the charity. Inadvertently, she has set up the company on a monthly cycle, too. They have monthly drives to gather supplies, and they distribute these the following week, 'Like in the Give phase!' she exclaimed.

🖤 During the Take phase, Gabby uses her power to be an effective campaigner by lobbying government officials about making periods better for women in need. She uses this energy when she really has to dig deep. 'I love that time of the month,' she said, leaning forward. 'I channel the fury.'

USE YOUR CRYSTAL VISIONS FOR GOOD

This isn't the time to start new projects; it's time to let go so you are free to do it all again. But first you must make a clean sweep and prepare for your biological verge pick-up (remember, I talked about this in the Dream phase; see page 103). Actual verge pick-up, where you leave your old furniture, etc., on the kerb for collection, usually happens once a year, and I either realise when it's too late and have to wait another year or I remember at 6 am the morning of, in which case I fly into the shed in a panic, torch in hand, looking for crap to go on the side of the road. Those lone forgotten legs from a foosball table, a snapped surfboard, a cracked flowerpot — I look at everything through an uber-critical lens and think, *Is this shit? Is that shit? Is it ALL actually shit? Should I just throw everything out and go to IKEA and start a new life?* This is a metaphor for how you can feel now. This is the work of this phase. To wade up to your waist in the muck.

Along with your endometrial lining, you can let go of whatever else it is that you don't need. You must make emotional room. It's out with the old and in with the new, and everything is up for scrutiny, including:

💜 emotional baggage

💜 mental strain

💜 any feeling about yourself that makes you feel smaller

LET IT ALL GO. This need for elimination is normal, and it will come every month. So invite it in like an old friend and make time for it. A few days into your Take phase, why not sit down with a cup of tea/hot chocolate and a pen and paper, and make a list of things to get rid of? Don't be horrified by this urge to purge, this is the natural time to look over at what you have left and decide whether you want to take it into a new month, or lighten your load and be free of it.

It's pretty incredible that we have this process of renewal built into our actual brains and wombs so that every month we get to start again and feel brand new. Do some writing, brainstorming or just a general stocktake of any feelings that are weighing you down: is there anything left unfinished or unsaid? Anything you want to get done before your Dream phase, when you go into your winter and *really* let go? Have a look at your last week of tracking for insights. Follow your footsteps in the snow.

Whether you make time for it or not, this process begs to be undertaken and is less enjoyable the longer you put it off. If you haven't had the time to consider the crap status of your current situation on the eve of chuck-out day (when your period starts), facing the crap all at once at the eleventh hour can be overwhelming and just *ARGH*. Get in early.

CLAIM YOUR FEELINGS

After looking at the world and your life through such a critical lens, sometimes what you are left with is powerful and intense, and it feels like the truth. Sometimes it's ugly, and looking at it in the eye is confronting. Then comes the pressure to minimise.

How many times have you heard someone say, 'Oh, it's just my hormones'? How many times have you sucked the air to the back of your top teeth in exasperation and said that to yourself?

This is the point at which your heightened sensitivity to whatever crap you've actually been putting up with all month leads your body to say, 'No, enough already. *STOP.*' How I wish I had listened to my inner voice as a teenager instead of rationalising my feelings away. Silencing our intuition sets us up for self-doubt (at any time in the cycle).

Part of why this phase is so challenging is because the break in the weather can be problematic for those around you, maybe even more so than it is for you. If someone is being a genuine asshole to you, you are more likely to notice it now. This can be particularly confronting for the person behaving like an asshole. If they try to insult you by blaming your hormones ('Are you on your *period* or something?'), don't take it personally. Their intention is to shift the focus away from them and what might have legitimately been a source of discontent for you, and that question is intended to minimise the issue. It always strikes me as doubly stupid because the person saying it is so ill-informed that they think you feel shitty purely because you are bleeding. As if that could be as bad as putting up with asshole behaviour.

It's not *just* your hormones.

No, doofus, it's you.

The clash and clang that you can feel here is the incongru-ence between what's going on *inside* you versus how you feel you should behave in the world. Psychologists call this 'emotional dissonance', and basically it means that pretending to be some-thing you aren't or feeling something that you don't can make you feel bonkers. When you feel out of sync and frustrated with how you *actually* feel and how you feel you *should* feel, the risk for catastrophe (when no one else can see your inner barometer) is dangerously high. It's a big fat lie that rankles us to the core.

I'm not suggesting that we should completely give in to our dominant feelings at every opportunity or lose our tempers and inflict our suffering on others because, of course, having to reg-ulate emotions is a normal part of being a grown-up human. I'm just saying that suppressing emotions is exhausting; it makes a difficult situation harder, and robs us of the benefits of this phase.

IDENTIFY SOME TRUTH BOMBS

Perhaps you've been calmly negotiating an insidious situation for three weeks, coming at it from all different angles and turning yourself into a pretzel as you work your way around it. Now your inner voice says, *Hey there. This is not okay. For real, it sucks.*

So, what to do with these truth bombs? The urge to act on them can be overpowering.

When you uncover a truth bomb, take a deep breath. They need be handled with care or they can blow up in your face. If you are premenstrual and something is giving you the shits, don't stew over it. Don't turn yourself into a salty, crunchy human pretzel. Spending too much of your Take power on things you can't control is like using holy water to clean the toilet. Shift your powerful focus to paper, and write down anything that feels big or true, then park it until your Dream phase rolls around. Later, when your body is slow and soft and letting go, you can revisit these truth bombs and uncover the most truth (there's a step-by-step guide to running these through your Dream filter in Chapter 4). This is not the right time/phase to act on these truth bombs, it's simply the time to see them.

If you are a natural campaigner, then by all means, channel the fury and use it. Imagine an army of premenstrual teenagers at a climate-change rally — this is the power that we need in the world. There is injustice everywhere, and you should feel angry when you see the way people are persecuted for their culture, sexuality or religion, or kept impoverished, and at the way the planet is being ravaged. Learn about it, name it, channel your rage and speak up about what you are seeing because we need women and girls to take control and call out the crap. Right now you are particularly able to take on the tigers and *win*. But as Maya Angelou said so wisely, 'Don't allow bitterness to eat you up.' We need you to be present and whole so that you can make changes when you are able. We don't want to see you half-eaten.

MY TRIP TO THE PMS ROADSHOW, BY KOPANO

Kopano is a gin-and-tonic-loving musician who makes synth-pop music. This is her story.

There are days that truly test the female spirit, and I was experiencing what felt like the worst of them all. Not only was I PMS-ing HARD, but the world had also decided to throw whatever it had at me the night of a gig I played at a bar called Jack Rabbit Slims.

I had a sold-out show to play and was really looking forward to it, but trouble began when my guitarist told me he'd double booked himself and had a show with his rock band. To top it off I had the worst period pains, and he told me this on the day of the show.

I arrived for a sound check unprepared for the technical changes I had to make on account of missing a guitarist. The sound guy was unsympathetic, and yet again I felt the humiliation of being 'another woman who didn't know what she was doing'. My god, I was bloated, angry and in emotional pain, embarrassed and feeling peak premenstrual madness, but I popped some Nurofen and tried to make the most of my night.

The world wasn't done with me yet.

At midnight, we were ready to load out but I couldn't find my keyboard. My anxiety heightened, and I was paranoid that another band had taken it. I couldn't think straight I was so stressed about it, and then, at 2 am, I was relieved to find that my keyboard and case had been handed in by someone who found them at the local park in the bushes (yes, you read that right). I opened the case to check that the keyboard was okay and was shocked to find that it was filthy and my case was full of dirt, soil and rocks. What. The (actual). Hell?

Well that was it. I was officially done — with my band and myself. I spent the car ride home bawling my eyes out. Was I being overdramatic? It felt like a sign. I went home to seek refuge in bed but lay awake until after 3 am with a premenstrual head-ache for my troubles.

A few days later, I was at Lucy Peach's show *My Greatest Period Ever.* I went with the mindset that my period was just a big bitch that I wanted to leave behind. Yet Lucy's storytelling, songs and the atmosphere she created for the crowd truly shifted me. When she called for someone who had had the worst week with their premenstrual self, you better believe I flipped the bird hard in response. She got me on stage to share my story, rewarded me with a cape and allowed me to let it all out.

It was so good to vent; it was fun. I may have even had a small cry. I was grateful to know that I wasn't alone in my premenstrual anger. Having that experience made me realise that perhaps my period wasn't the enemy after all; it was a friend. After that, I decided that I never wanted to experience that again in my creativity and artistry. I knew I was ready for a change. My feelings were valid, and Lucy helped me come to terms with that.

PS. Kopano has since embarked on a solo career where she presses all of the buttons and is striving to become the artist she wants to be. She is going great.

MAKE SOMETHING YOU LOVE

There is something pretty special about creating when you are in this space of free fall because not only are your senses sharper, but you also give less of a shit about what anyone else might think and you are more easily able to commit to your purest intentions. That fizzy, prickly energy is desperate for an outlet, so make the most of it.

Writing, gardening, bridge building, singing, dancing, cooking, sculpting, crafting . . . Absolutely. But the washing? It can wait.

'I'm just not arty,' some people insist, but, as Elizabeth Gilbert writes in her book *Big Magic,* 'We've been creating art for longer than we have been developing tools — it's in our nature.' This book is a good one for you if you feel that you are waiting for permission to be creative. Just do something that makes you feel the most like you, especially when you get that *Fark!* feeling.

If you can train your critical self to zip it while you open up your creative channels, the rewards can be great. I guarantee that with an emptying cup and not much to give, you will feel a lot less prickly if you can channel some of this premenstrual energy into something you love; everything you say will be less likely to come out like a lion's roar. You might even be quite thrilled by what you discover.

I used to waste this phase trying to fix people (okay, boy-friends who were probably mostly fine) or on cleaning things such as skirting boards *with a toothbrush*, and I'd feel so put upon when demands were made of me like 'Could you please pass the salt?' or 'Have you seen my sock/keys/phone?' Requests like these were (and sometimes still are) enough to send me over the edge.

Then, when I first started learning about the menstrual cycle in *The Optimized Woman* by Miranda Gray, I realised that I could also use this phase to make music — Miranda calls this time 'the creative phase', straight up. During the Dream phase I like mulling over lyrics more. During the Do phase I get organised and schedule rehearsals or make plans for recording sessions and future shows. In the Give phase I like to plan co-writing sessions with other people, rehearsals with my band, or go and see other bands play.

But it's in the Take phase that I am always the most creatively productive. I know now that this is when I'm most likely to be able to write a good song (and some crap ones, too). Most of all, I know that if I don't spend some of my Take power doing what I love, I will feel crappy — like I've ignored a precious part of myself. I also know that the precious part gets mighty pissed off if I do this, and she'll take it out on those in close proximity. 'How dare you deny me?!' she roars.

'Okay, okay, okay!' I placate her, sometimes just in time, by reaching for my guitar and singing from my darkest places.

Look for a seed of goodness, then make something from it with your hands or your voice or your body, and stitch it in. Being creative is a protective practice. It hooks you into your deepest self so the noise of the world melts away.

It's quite good to choose an activity that isn't too precious, so if you do 'stuff it up' it doesn't actually matter. This is not the time to be learning how to leadlight under pressure.

Sarah, who works in my local café, spoke to me after reading the sign on my laptop that says, 'Hi, ask me about the book I'm writing about periods.' She designs and makes her own clothes, and she told me that she's creative all the time, but that it's actually hardest for her to make clothes when she's premenstrual. 'I like sewing with fabulous material,' she says, 'and if I f%ck it up, it's a disaster.'

Sarah went on to tell me about something that had happened the previous day (and she was still clearly quite furious about it). She'd been all set to make a pair of pink-silk wide-leg palazzo pants. She'd measured the silk, cut up the pieces and started stitching. They were perfect, and she imagined herself with bright red lipstick and that luxurious pink silk snug against her lovely bum. But it wasn't to be. She'd made them *back to front* and the zip that should have been at the back was now at the front, 'perfectly drawing attention to my fanny'.

Thankfully, one can always make mistakes and then simply cut up the fabric to make something else, which is what Sarah did. And after our chat, she proceeded to tell the man sitting next to me in the corner about the perils of PMS and why men need to be more understanding. I explained the graph of the phases to him and he said, 'Wait, this is just like how I check the weather before I go surfing. But hang on, why would my partner not talk about this?'

Well, as we discussed in the history of PMS, no one wants to talk about these feelings unless they know they are safe to. So, to any males reading this (you're awesome), make sure the women and girls in your life feel safe expressing themselves to you, and know you are doing a good service for humanity. Consider making them dinner while they make something else that makes them happy. Measure twice, cut once. Everyone wins.

You only get twelve of these phases a year, so give yourself permission to make a mess, to be a mess and see what you come up with. I feel a bit ripped off if I miss out on a chance to make something in this phase. What might I have made? Joining a band helped me channel my biggest, most painful feelings through the breakdown of my first marriage, and speaking truth to them and singing them made me feel like it wasn't all in my head. It made me feel heard, even if I was the only one listening.

The other great thing — possibly the greatest thing — about doing something creative that you *love* while you're premenstrual is that not only will you avoid spending this energy trying to fix people or criticise yourself, BUT YOU WILL ACTUALLY GET BETTER AT YOUR CREATIVE PURSUIT, TOO.

Sophie was eleven when she first came to see *My Greatest Period Ever*. She sat wide-eyed through the show and said little afterwards. But in the following months, she started to incorporate what she'd learned into her own creative practice; she spent time drawing when she was in her Take phase and started telling her mum that she'd be unavailable for a few hours. Sophie would go to her room, shut the door, put on her favourite playlist and lose herself with paper and pencils. And you know something? Three years later, at fourteen, her drawings are *really good*.

Being premenstrual is powerful, so take the power and run with it.

GO ALL-IN ON THE 'THING' YOU LOVE

Give yourself time and space not just to be creative in a regular way, but occasionally to back yourself and do something BIG. After I had a baby, I got brave and found 'my thing'. Music became my best friend, and I enjoyed it the most when I was premenstrual (still do). In hard times, this connection made me feel alive and, as any artist will attest, it's free therapy.

Years later, I was booked as a support act for a folk band on a small tour of Australia's eastern states. The schedule meant that there were six days between two chunks of shows, and I was debating how to spend them. Should I come home to Perth and back again or stay in Melbourne and have a great time? I checked my calendar and saw that I'd be in my Take phase for those six days. *Hmmm, this changes things,* I thought. I'd been journalling for a long time about how I felt throughout my cycle, and I wanted to distil all of this material into four songs about my experiences of the phases. I booked a cabin in the forest.

It was the middle of autumn (pretty perfect in my premenstrual condition), and I stayed in a town called Bright where there were majestic trees in various states of undress, with masses of red and orange and golden leaves lining the streets and surrounding my cabin. I went off to the local shop to get stocked up on supplies then settled in and lit the fire. I set up my recording space and cooked a ginormous pot of dhal that kept me fed (and tooting) through the week.

Every day I would write and sing and play, taking breaks for food and walks in the leaves, and then at 8 pm I would record what I had done. I did this every day for four days, and on the fifth day I rewarded myself with a day out in Bright and an op-shop tour. (Bright is heaven for op-shoppers because so many old people go there to retire and then at some point they die, leaving masses of crocheted items and pretty teacups, so I was in my element.)

I left Bright with a crocheted pink tea cosy that looked like it was made of vulvas, four new songs and more faith in my Take phase than I'd ever had before. I cannot recommend an experience like this enough. If you have always wanted some time alone to create and you already have what you need to get going, plan a 'making week' to coincide with your Take phase. There is no better way to befriend this power.

PLAY TO YOUR STRENGTHS AT WORK

My friend Ghazal is a clinical psychologist. She works in human resources, managing of a team of psychologists. Over the last three years, she has cultivated a team culture where the menstrual cycle is freely spoken of. Ghazal says that while team members may be unsure about this at first, as psychologists they understand the benefits of a cycle-centric work space.

When calling out a general request for help across the open-plan office, she says it isn't uncommon for a few hands to go up accompanied by brief comments such as, 'Day 28 here, just no.' Everyone nods in sympathy, and requests are diverted elsewhere for the time being. It makes sense because it works.

CONSTRUCTIVE DESTRUCTION

When you feel that the familiar prickle of the Take phase is starting to work its way under your skin, channel it to let go in all areas of your life. Have a good wardrobe cull or a desk clear out, delete photos that take up valuable space or prune that bougainvillea as a productive way to feel vicious. I couldn't care less what the neighbours think as I grunt, howl and exclaim while chopping off a big, thorny branch. I hack and swear, sweaty and triumphant.

Any work that needs final editing is a good job for now, too, as you have a particularly ruthless eye. This is also a favourite time to write without any real attachment to the outcome. It just feels good to pull at the edges of words and push them into line. I daren't waste *all* of my Take power on the garden because that's what my body gave me and I need to make something of it.

STAND UP FOR YOURSELF

If someone crosses your boundaries in a not-okay way, wherever you happen to be — at work or in the rest of your life — you have a right to feel violated. And if your premenstrual self starts squaring up in the corner and if you feel safe enough to do so, let her be your ally.

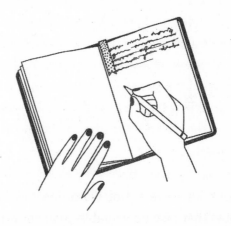

CHALLENGES IN THE TAKE PHASE

Challenges. The word conjures up an image of something fairly manageable to be surmounted, with a bit of effort. Like jumping over a small ditch. Challenges? In a world where women have been under the thumb of the patriarchy, the list is longer than any lifetime. Challenges? The ancient woman inside of us all laughs so hard that she nearly chokes on her own tongue. Then she draws a breath.

We are still subordinated and denied opportunity, education and positions of power. Women of colour are more likely to be paid less and to work twice as hard in jobs that invite judgment such as sex work and factory work. Women face challenges at the sink, in the streets, in courtrooms, in doctor's surgeries, and while carrying babies in and on their bodies. They are preyed upon in the dark, in broad daylight and in their homes, if they have them.

In Australia, older women who sacrificed the income opportunities and superannuations enjoyed by their husbands to work unpaid in the home are now the fastest-growing group facing homelessness. For Indigenous women, the hurdles are even higher, especially in Australia where systemic racism and inequality are still rife.

HOT, BURNING ANGER

No matter where you are or what your life looks like, this week everything hard about your life can be so much harder. This week, your ability to put up with crap is all but abolished. My lovely mother says that this is the phase when she feels most like 'ramming into cars' and 'biting her water glass'.

Sometimes life conspires in such a way that every annoying thing that could possibly happen does — all at once. As a result, you might feel like barking at anyone who comes within 3 metres of you just because of the way they breathe or fail to replace a toilet roll or send three 'friendly reminder' emails in one day. Fact: you will be more likely to feel this if you (or your circumstances) have denied you adequate time and space for self-care.

If the upcoming menstrual Dream phase is defined by having zero f%cks to give, then during the premenstrual phase, your f%cks are fading fast. You might have a precious few left. When you're expected to use those precious dwindling resources on trivial matters, the rage can be real. Worse if you are being mistreated.

Every slight and extra task that you do now is mentally noted: someone else's toothpaste residue worried off with your finger, the piss splatters on the floor. No one tells you how much of your life will be spent wiping! You can go to university for ten years (if you're lucky), but you will still wipe up the evidence of other people. If you are lucky enough to have a home and you've chosen to populate it with tiny versions of yourself, there will be considerable wiping. And with a few to zero f%cks left to give, every wipe can feel like an insult.

In the biography *Margaret Olley: Far from a still life*, about the life of the Australian painter, who held over 90 solo exhibitions, author Meg Stewart recounts Olley's approach to domesticity — perhaps one we'd be wise to emulate: 'I've never liked housework. I get by doing little chores when I feel like them, in between paintings. Who wants to chase dust all their life? You can spend your whole lifetime cleaning the house. I like watching the patina grow. If the house looks dirty, buy another bunch of flowers, is my advice.'

During this phase, if the dinner is shit and you made it, only you can say it's shit. If you make a joke about it then other people (who did nothing to help make it) may laugh, but then they'd better say something that ameliorates your original comment, and they would be wise to follow up their comment with a second comment that expresses sincere gratitude that someone actually made food at all. I feel this practice is fairly self-explanatory.

One premenstrual evening, I laughed at how royally I'd managed to ruin each element of the meal. The sweet potatoes were burned, the eggplant was chewy and undercooked, and everyone prodded the meal without any comment. I felt like flicking salad at them. 'Well, the salad is nice, Mum,' my son said brightly. (The salad was a bag of lettuce with oil and vinegar on it.)

'Yes,' I said, 'eat it all.'

LOVED ONES AND THE SUPER-CRITICAL LENS

If not carefully managed, the poo-coloured glasses phenomenon can take its toll on relationships, which is why I feel this tender area requires its own section.

You see, at the root of your Take phase power is the deep, unbridled need to be with your own magic and to take care of your own self. Self-love is key to any healthy relationship, menstrual cycle or not, and Richard and I felt so strongly about this that it featured in our wedding vows: 'I promise to honour and cherish my own heart so that I may be able to honour and cherish yours.' We straight-up acknowledged in front of our friends and family that without self-love, our relationship is screwed. We made a promise to each other, and mine was wrapped around the knowledge that at different times of the month, I have different needs. It's up to him to respond (or not), but it's up to me to communicate openly. This doesn't mean that we are always perfectly in sync, but we're less likely to react to each other and end up in a shit spiral without knowing why.

I know two young women, Bella and Orla, who are both eighteen. They have read parts of this book in the interest of quality control because they are OBSESSED with their menstrual cycles, so much so that they dress accordingly. The last time they visited me for tea, chocolate and period chats, Orla was in her Do phase in a fantastic lime-green satin crop top with matching flares. Bella was deep in her Take phase and wearing a long black flowing dress that she'd tucked into her knickers.

We spoke about their generation and the young men they knew, and Bella said, 'I just can't imagine being with a guy who didn't know where I was in my cycle.'

'Hallelujah,' I said. And I felt that same thought with every fibre of my being because I would like all women to be unable to imagine that. However . . .

Getting to a place where that is the reality for all women will take time. It took me several significant relationships and a good one with myself before I met someone who understands and celebrates the fact that I am cyclical. Richard has a fairly good idea of which phase I am in, but the onus is still on me to say, 'Babe, I need time/space/help/hugs/a wine/a whinge/a bath/etc.' And if I do this, chances are my needs will be (mostly) met.

He knows the ebbs and flows; he understands that if I am supported and able to give myself what I need, he'll be out of the firing line and I'll be the best partner I can be — this is what he wants for me, too. We will both be happier.

Openly stating what I need is also a reminder to him to share his needs with me. (Bearing in mind that bigger requests are best received in T + 10 days, or requested from someone else.)

But even with good support, small things can still feel catastrophic. Sometimes, shit happens. Especially when there are small people in the equation who don't have the same emotional sensitivity as a loving partner (and can't wipe their own bums).

As children, my sister and I knew our tender-hearted mother loved us dearly. Sometimes she'd even let us sleep in bed with her. But there were times (and I'm sure they were in this phase for her particularly) that if we wriggled just one too many times she'd say, in a voice with no emotion, 'Get. Out.' We knew to go without fuss. We got out. And now we say it to our own children.

It's normal to feel less patient now. If the thought of playing yet another session of LEGO or shops makes your brain begin to pulsate — give yourself a break. If it's raining, you're late and you want to throw the small shoe that needs to be put on the small foot — give yourself a break. 'Yes, you need to wear your seatbelt.' 'No, you can't have Smarties for breakfast, and I don't care that your sister looked at you.' Give yourself a break. There's a lot of pressure to be endlessly accommodating to our children, and to feel guilty when we aren't. But you are only human, and so is the rest of the world.

Your child needs to know that not everyone will understand them and treat them as though they are the centre of the universe. What better way for them to learn this than when their mother is premenstrual? You are teaching them boundaries, how to recognise when someone has nothing to give, and how important and worthy of love their mother is. We all get a turn.

Arrange a play date that you can reciprocate when you are in the Give phase. Precook some dinners, or, if you share the cooking, take this week off. Otherwise it's a boiled egg and some Weetbix. Start communicating your needs to your children as soon as they are able to understand words: 'Mummy is very tired today and will be tomorrow, too. I love it when you help.' If you have a boy like I do, one day they'll not only be tying their own laces but also be saying, 'Sounds like you need a cup of tea, Mum.' Then they'll make you one (and you might even cry a few tears of gratitude). When you care for yourself, your children learn to do the same.

If you find yourself having a Take tanty, pause. Are you holding your breath? Could you stop for ten minutes? Maybe you could find a moment in nature and someone else could do the wiping.

Just as you've been tuning in to any pain during your period and listening to your body, listen to your anger. You can work out the source of it by checking in and asking yourself these questions:

🖤 Could I be more supported?

🖤 Have I said yes to things I regret?

🖤 Am I sweating the small things?

🖤 Am I feeling powerless about something?

🖤 What could I do to feel more in control?

🖤 Do I feel pressured?

🖤 How can I make more breathing space for myself?

🖤 Is there a way to reframe what is currently challenging me?

🖤 Am I dealing with asshole behaviour?

Don't feel like you need to be a positive Polly and see genuine poo through rose-tinted glasses, but if there is a different way of considering something that feels better, then reach for that.

Write down how you feel, and try not to worry about the details. Actively divert all flights of your attention to things that make you feel good — sunshine, hugs and chocolate. And have a good cry if you need to, or a howl. Then do something you love.

IF YOU DO LOSE YOUR COOL, REGROUP

Losing your cool is usually something that happens when you've been 'holding on'. If you do snap and feel like, *Everyone is taking everything from me. I have nothing,* then maybe you gave too much away in your Give phase. Or maybe you *are* surrounded by selfish idiots. Either way, if you don't have enough energy for even the bare necessities, then you will be much more likely to snap. If you hold on to tension — or to a feeling, or to something that is better out than in — for too long, before you know it, some (possibly inconsequential and not that annoying) thing will tip you over the edge and *ARGH! Everything is shit!*

If you are in mid-wobble right now . . .

1. **Firstly, forgive yourself.** This is called being human. The art is in how you recover afterwards. This is what Miles Davis was talking about when he supposedly said, 'It's not the note you play that's the wrong note; it's the note you play afterwards that makes it right or wrong.' He was talking in the context of jazz, and how the music you play *after* the 'bum note' says more about who you are. The same is true here. Don't freak out, don't admit defeat. Make it work, be as gracious as you can and, above all, preserve the self.

2. **Breathe.** Drop your shoulders, have a yawn and relax that jaw. Make fists and shake your hands out and breathe. I mean *really* breathe. When we're feeling prickly, it's as though there is a multitude of tight springs filling our body, ready to pop out and poke something. So take the kind of

breath that will give your whole body much-needed oxygen and make everything a little bit looser. I know it's boring, but just do it and keep doing it. Take a deep breath, and now an even deeper one. You need to thoroughly oxygenate that brain of yours before you give it any new information.

3. **Do some damage control.** Take some time out. Let off steam in the privacy of your own space. Maybe you can't move to the country, start a herb farm and home school your children, but could you go for a walk and sniff some flowers or watch a sunset? Write down what happened if you want to revisit it later. Soften your heart and appeal to the best in those around you, say sorry if you need to and get on with your life. Alternatively, don't wait for an apology before getting on with your life, either.

4. **Try a little more self-care next month.** If you spend every single scrap of goodness in your Give phase, you'll enter Take with nothing left to actually *take* for yourself, so be mindful of this. If you don't quite get it right, there's always next month to aim for a nicer time for yourself. Your Take phase will benefit as a result — it all adds up and it's here that we pay for it.

Of house cleaning, author Clarissa Pinkola Estés writes in her book, *Women Who Run With the Wolves*: 'It never comes to an end. Perfect way to stop a woman. A woman must be careful to not allow over-responsibility (or over-respectability) to steal her necessary creative rests, riffs, and raptures. She simply must put her foot down and say no to half of what she believes she "should" be doing. Art is not meant to be created in stolen moments only.' See the dirty windows or the unfinished email and let your eyes glaze over. There are more important things, and you are one of them.

Lots of people can relate to the feeling of the 'penny dropping' once their bleed begins. *Oh. So that's why that happened.* Maybe you felt extra sensitive or irritable about something, and just before your period came it really, really got to you. When I'm in my Take phase, small things can feel big, and big things feel absolutely epic. There are two obvious ways to deal with these irritations and grievances. The first is to blame yourself and think, *Well, it's just me and my stupid hormones.* The second is to completely blame someone/something else and think, *It's all them.* Unless you are an actual saint surrounded by numbskulls (look, it is possible), then the truth is usually somewhere in the middle. But if you're really stuck, the upcoming Dream phase will help you work out the balance.

WHEN TO GET HELP

The intensity of this time is different for each of us and how it affects you depends largely on your hormone sensitivity. While some people might not notice it too much, others notice the hell out of it. The shadow can be overwhelming and the symptoms devastating. Feeling this all alone and thinking it's 'all in your head' can be absolutely crushing.

Don't despair, there are things you can do and natural treatments you can explore. In *Period Repair Manual*, Dr Lara Briden explains that we now know that, at least for some of the time, the symptoms of PMS and PMDD are exacerbated by histamines; these are found in most of our tissues, stored in cells called mast cells that are a part of our immune system. They are released as part of the inflammatory response we see with allergies that cause itchiness and congestion, mucus production, etc.

To alleviate PMS symptoms such as anxiety, fatigue, head-aches and achiness, explore anti-inflammatory nutritional strategies such as eating dairy-free and taking supplements of vitamin B6 and magnesium.*

If, after all of this understanding and self-care, this phase continues to be your least favourite and you are suffering and need help, then ask for it. Find a doctor, health practitioner, naturopath or someone who specialises in women's health and can give you the support you need. Even just a good friend can make all of the difference, but don't suffer in silence.

Look after your body, pay attention to your precious self and listen to what your deepest feelings are telling you. If you can stay mindful of your mood now, you'll be more likely to catch yourself before you get worked up and so tense that you get a doozie of a migraine. But sometimes they just happen.

If I'm in a stressful situation, or life is really busy and I've skidded into this phase on empty, I'm more likely to suffer intense physical symptoms. Every three months or so, I feel like I have been punched in the face with a migraine, and it builds and builds until I bleed. My skin feels like it has an electric charge, and my fingertips actually tingle. The worst thing is I know I need to breathe and relax but it's too late for that now. My jaw's wired

*Period Repair Manual *goes into this in more detail.*

Period Queen

shut, teeth clamp together, and every muscle in my head and face feels like it has passed the point of no return. My eyeballs ache, my temples throb, and there's nothing to do but surrender up the self-care and wait.

It's your body's way of putting you down to rest, whether you like it or not.

WHERE THE HELL IS MY PERIOD?

A period going AWOL can lead to the longest Take phase ever. Sometimes your cycle is considerably longer. Why? Lots of reasons, but the main one is stress. If you are holding on, your body will, too. And the stress doesn't have to be negative, it can also be positive stress, as in you just got too dang excited in the Give phase and forgot to calm down. Do whatever you can to find balance and peace. Soften yourself so that your body knows it's safe to let go.

If you are hoping your period won't come because you want to be pregnant, the wait can be unbearable, or just annoying — as can the expense of pregnancy tests that claim they can detect pregnancy several days before your period is due.

Here's a tip: remember that your temperature increased after ovulation, and it will stay high until just before your period comes. So take your morning temperature, and don't bother with a pregnancy test if it drops down to pre-ovulatory levels, as this means you will bleed very soon. If you are pregnant, your temperature will stay high.

PREPARiNG TO DREAM

If you get some spotting this week, consider it a warning — the final snooze before the internal alarm goes off and you enter the cave of dreams to rest. Use the remaining time wisely.

I use various scaffolding strategies to prepare and support myself in each of the phases. Here are some nice things to do just before your period arrives.

- 🖤 Stock up on dark chocolate and avocados.
- 🖤 Get re-usable pads and knickers organised.
- 🖤 Schedule in some quiet bleeding time.
- 🖤 Change the sheets and tidy the bedroom to make it a restful, peaceful space.
- 🖤 Wash your dressing gown so when you start bleeding you feel snuggly and divine.
- 🖤 Wash your hair (especially if you've gotten wild and filthy).
- 🖤 Tick some last boxes so that you can rest more later when you need to. If you've procrastinated, this is a window for blitzing before slowing down. If you can kick a few more goals before you bleed, you might feel like you've really earned the right to slow down and rest.
- 🖤 Make a period cake that no one else is allowed to eat. This idea came from my sweet friend Uma Spender, a yoga teacher and expert in celebrating the feminine. She makes a

cake (preferably something rich, nourishing and chocolatey), puts it in a tin, hides it from everyone else and then nibbles away at it during her Dream phase.

💜 If you have cramps, 'period flu' or a migraine, try to make friends with your pain. Don't push against it. This is the time to really dial up the self-love strategies (which you can borrow from the Dream phase chapter). Know that on a deep, cellular level this fiery part of you is just as worthy of approval, care and time.

💜 Meditation is preventative medicine for the Take phase. You don't need to make it complicated, just relax your jaw and imagine the space between your eyes as smooth and soft. Breathe into it deeply, and vow to notice when you are shallow breathing. Try using a mantra or a guided meditation.

💜 If you feel sad, go for a walk. And if you go for a walk and you don't feel better, keep walking a bit further. If the next day you still feel sad and moving your body isn't shifting that, and nothing is working, then just walk again anyway because I reckon it takes a minimum of three days to walk out the sads/overwhelm. But I always have to learn that again and again. Three days.

💜 NOTHING. In writing this book I have enjoyed writing from all the phases for different reasons. There are ways and means around everything, but for me the last day before my period truly arrives is the time that requires as much, if not *more,* rest and relaxation as when it actually arrives. If you simply cannot do the thing — the conversation, the assignment, the task requiring your brain — but you have a looming deadline and some pressure, then your pressurised body can respond badly. 'ARGH!' all your nerve endings will scream with indignation. 'You can't make me!'

My advice: keep some rubber room in your diary and don't overbook yourself. Particularly if you are a last-minute, wing-it type of person, allow yourself a day of exemption.

LIMINAL SPACE

A liminal space is a threshold — a doorway between what was and what is next. If you consider the Give phase and the peak of your ovulatory power as 'what was', the Take phase is the liminal space through which you move towards 'what is next' — the deeper, more introspective time of menstruation. After the full mind and body reset in the Dream phase, your power is restored. But we have to be broken down before we can be rebuilt.

If that sounds overly dramatic, consider your womb lining: you spent weeks perfecting it, but now your body will tear it down before you begin anew. Males don't experience this process in the same way. Feminine embodiment coach Breeda McKibbin says that's why they jump off bridges into rivers and want to be in fast cars — they seek to create a liminal space.

As you approach yours, you might feel twitchy. Change is afoot. What is there to hold on to? Will you be the same when you emerge? What might you lose? A friend? An eye? Your sanity? You'll need to be your greatest ally while you face your harshest critic.

For many people, the emotional and physical twitchiness intensifies exponentially until the final moment before the blood comes. It can be uncomfortable and painful but we must pass through it, even when only kicking the door down will do. We teeter across two worlds for a moment before a leap of faith through the darkest parts of ourselves. And this is where we meet the most potential for transformation. When you are premenstrual, you are not crazy, *you are not crazy*, YOU ARE NOT CRAZY, and if you get to know and fall in love with who you are this week, even if much of society doesn't understand her yet, you'll discover silver linings and hidden treasures. As you free-fall, shake off your old skin. Trust that you will land safely back at the beginning of yourself, and release a full body sigh of surrender and relief: 'Ahhhh.' Letting go and landing on familiar ground.

Every month, by hook or by crook, we forge a new path. If you channel the Take power and scaffold yourself, you will experience the triumph that is your reward.

LiFTiNG THE CURSE

At her first bleeding a woman meets her power.
In her bleeding years she practises it.
At menopause she becomes it.

Yesterday, on Day 30, I did not feel like surrendering. 'Probably just tired,' I huffed. But there was something else asking to be seen. I turned over in bed to face Richard. It wasn't him. I searched my body and found it: fear. Even though I've been doing this work — this period preaching — for years, I've only recently felt the backlash. And as much as I love doing this work, I wish it wasn't needed and that pride and safety in our bodies was something we felt for all of our lives.

With the sliver of a new moon peeking through a crack in the thunderclouds, I confessed to Richard. 'I'm afraid.' He held an arm out and I rolled into it. I sobbed until my face was wet against his chest. And as I lay there, I remembered something my dear friend Mama Kin had said: 'The bigger the light, the bigger the shadow. But the shadow? It's nothing without the light.'

This morning the thunderclouds gave way to heavy rain. I hid my laptop under the bed and stretch-danced with hand weights for an entire Stevie Nicks album, laughing and singing until I could hear my breath and my cheeks were pink. And then, like a red carpet, my period came.

Ahh. There you are . . .

So now I have a hot water bottle and a mug of hot chocolate and it's just you and me with this last bite of pie. Before I go, there are a few things left to say.

I thought about calling this book *Our Greatest Period Ever*. But, really, it's not even about periods; it's about this period in time. There's no denying we are in the midst of a collective move towards restoring balance and equality, but I would be remiss to suggest that smooth sailing awaits so long as you simply celebrate your cycle. The truth is that to really lift this curse, we need help.

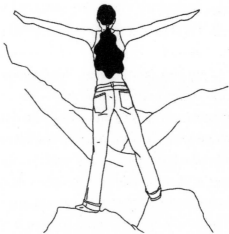

DEAR MEN . . .

You are key. If you are a man reading this, hi and thank you. We can't do this without you. Join us. Celebrate with us, ask questions and help us to feel safe. Trust that the benefits of supporting your partners, colleagues, sisters, mothers and friends throughout the month also extend to you. If a potential partner mentions their cycle to you, see this as an invitation. Embrace it.

If you're a father, your support is needed now more than ever. When you love your daughter for each of her four ways, you support her to know her whole self and to connect to her deepest heart and greatest potential. Hold her close in her Dream phase and encourage her to slow down. Build her up in her Do phase to be brave. In her Give phase, celebrate her. Help her fill her cup with self-love and confidence. Allow her plenty of space in her Take phase, and don't take anything too personally. She needs to feel out the boundaries for herself and push against them; you are her container. Champion her power and welcome it. Show her how it feels when a man respects the life-giving qualities of her body. She might meet some that aren't ready.

POWER TO THE PERIOD

Just to be clear, I'm not saying you must talk about your cycle nonstop (unless you want to) in order to truly embrace your power, but imagine if you could say how you actually feel on any given day, and why. Imagine if people asked not just *how* are you, but *where* are you in your cycle. Imagine if they listened.

There's nothing like being heard to alleviate an ache. A lovely way to support your cycle is to participate in a circle with others. The Red Tent movement is about this very thing: women making spaces to come together for ceremony, to share stories, to rest and connect. You can join one or start your own. It doesn't need to be complicated; it's not something you can get wrong. As my young friend Orla suggested, it could be as simple as going to the beach with friends, lighting a stick of incense and sitting in a circle with a box of hot chips in the middle.

Anything you do to stitch in your power and cultivate pride is an act of love. On the other hand, some people, are mortified that we would dare talk about our cycles. They think it's gross and weird. I think it's pretty weird that we're made of the same stuff as stars and lions and share nearly 60 per cent of the same genetic material with a banana, but I don't let it stop me enjoying my life or use it as an excuse to stop anyone else from enjoying theirs. If you come across a negative attitude towards your cycle, turn on your heel and don't be deterred from being as fabulous as possible. Some people actually *are* bananas.

Let the shadows dance and turn, my friend, to the big red flashing light that is popping up all over the world like a beacon, as girls, women and menstruators everywhere say, **we are powerful**.

If you have a young girl or daughter in your life, the best way to teach her about her power and how to love her body in all its glory is to show her by example. How do you love yours? What words do you use to describe it? What small ceremonies do you have to honour the arrival of your own blood?

Whether it's a movie night, a chocolate bar, a day of rest or painting each other's toes — start a little tradition with her as soon as you can — it's a gift to both of you. Modelling how you honour your cycle in every phase will stand her in good stead to honour hers.

There are endless ways to create a rite of passage. When my friend Mama Kin knew her daughter Banjo's first period was imminent, she wrote a letter to Banjo's 'aunties' — women who'd been instrumental in her daughter's life. 'Banjo will bleed one day soon,' she wrote, 'and when she does, I want you all to speak to the power of this transition and chapter. What would you most like her to have or to know when her time comes? Start preparing a letter and a small gift. When she first bleeds, I will let you know to pop them in the post so we have them ready.'

When the second letter came some two years later, the women started sending small packages: a poem, a warm scarf, lavender oil, a treasured book, a lipstick, a playlist. And on the next full moon after her first period, Banjo, her aunties, some of her friends and their mothers met at the river with flasks of tea and tins of chocolate cake. They slipped into waiting canoes and paddled upstream, talking, singing, laughing and then quiet, carving through the water with long strokes in unison.

The moon rose ahead of them, throwing a staircase down onto the still waters. When they arrived at a grassy bank, they tied up their canoes and honoured Banjo with a ceremony. They formed a circle, and Banjo stood in the centre. When she turned to each of them, they put their hands on her shoulders and honoured her in whichever way they chose: with a funny memory, a dream for her future or acknowledgment of her gifts. After this, they sat together and Banjo shared how loved and held she felt.

If you don't have a daughter, treat your inner girl with this much love, too. Perhaps you are no longer a young woman but you still yearn to be celebrated. It's never too late to honour your cycle, wherever you find yourself.

One day, after months and years of practising in your own ways, you won't need your blood anymore to remind you of your power. At menopause you *become* your power, and we aren't the only creatures to live beyond our reproductive years and experience this. Grandmother orcas play a role much bigger than breeding: they are the wise ones — the keepers of knowledge. They guide the young, warning them of danger and singing songs about where the water is best and the fish most bountiful. Without them, young whales suffer, particularly the males — who die earlier. These matriarchs and the knowledge they pass on are essential to the survival of the pod. As are we. One day, you may be a grandmother (or old enough to be one), and your wisdom will help those that come after you.

NOW, iT'S YOUR TURN

Once you've met your powers and loved yourself all month long, you can never unknow that you are a period queen. It's not a title you earn, it just is. Written into your bones. You claim it with every step and every stride, every laugh and every cry.

As sure as the world turns on its axis, under the watchful eye of the moon, so do you on yours. As you reach towards the bright lights of who you are and who you want to be, this force is always with you. You carry it, and it carries you. Like every woman that came before you; it's in your blood: an unbroken thread that binds us all. Nature anointed you with a cycle, and its four hormonal phases are baked into your being: of who you are, and why, when and how you are.

Learn to surrender, to say yes to yourself and see the strength in your softness. Stay open to the gifts of each phase and cycle, and be curious and playful with whatever challenges or joys await. Your power ebbs and flows in rivers that unravel to reveal new mysteries and magic at every turn. Treasures left like perfect shells on a foamy shore — gifts from your tides. All the while you are guided and held with time for everything: a time to Dream, to Do, to Give and to Take. Each phase of your multifaceted self is a precious resource to be tasted, tested and held up as a triumph. Four unique ways to see the world and to move within it. Four ways to change it and to channel the deepest of desires.

Behold our power.

All hail the queens.

This is the beginning.

GREAT READS & REFERENCES

💜 *We are Dancing for You: Native feminisms & the revitalization of women's coming-of-age ceremonies* by Cutcha Risling Baldy

💜 *The Managed Body: Developing girls and menstrual health in the global south* by Chris Bobel

💜 *Period Repair Manual: Natural treatment for better hormones and better periods* by Dr Lara Briden

💜 *Women Who Run With the Wolves: Myths and stories of the wild woman archetype* by Clarissa Pinkola Estés

💜 *Fight Like a Girl* by Clementine Ford

💜 *Big Magic: Creative living beyond fear* by Elizabeth Gilbert

💜 *The Optimized Woman: Using your menstrual cycle to achieve success and fulfillment* by Miranda Gray

💜 *The Fifth Vital Sign: Master your cycles & optimize your fertility* by Lisa Hendrickson-Jack

💜 *Period Power: Harness your hormones and get your cycle working for you* by Maisie Hill

💜 *Blood Relations: Menstruation and the origins of culture* by Chris Knight

💜 *How To Be a Woman* by Caitlin Moran

💜 *Cunt: A declaration of independence* by Inga Muscio

💜 *Women's Bodies, Women's Wisdom: Creating physical and emotional health and healing* by Christiane Northrup

💜 *Her Blood is Gold: Awakening to the wisdom of menstruation* by Lara Owen

💜 *About Bloody Time: The menstrual revolution we have to have* by Karen Pickering and Jane Bennett

💜 *Wild Power: Discover the magic of your menstrual cycle and awaken the feminine path to power* by Alexandra Pope and Sjanie Hugo Wurlitzer

💜 *Brainstorm: The power and purpose of the teenage brain* by Daniel J. Siegel

💜 *The Great Cosmic Mother* by Monica Sjöö and Barbara Mor

💜 *Period. End of Sentence.* A documentary by Rayka Zehtabchi

SPECIAL THANKS

I am thankful. Firstly, to the custodians of the Whadjuk Noongar nation on whose boodja I live and work. It always was, and always will be, Aboriginal land. To my first menstrual mentor, Miranda Gray, for opening my eyes at just the right time, I am forever indebted. To Alexandra Pope and Sjanie Hugo Wurlitzer, pioneers of menstruality and co-directors of Red School, for creating a global community and welcoming me into it.

To Alan Gilrod for aiming me at theatre, and to Mia Freedman for leading me back to writing.

To the wonderful team at Murdoch Books for seeing the potential here and helping me hold it: my publisher Jane Morrow, Megan Pigott (who suggested me to Jane), Julie Mazur Tribe, Katie Bosher and Ngaio Parr. Thank you all for your powers!

To my expert contributors: Chris Bobel, Chris Knight, Robin Litvins Salter and especially Lara Briden and Peta Wright, for sharing your essential advice so generously. To those first readers and friends who gave invaluable feedback: Dan, Ellie, Isabella, Jane, Kim, Luke, Marianne, Michelle, Orla, Rachel, Reuben (infinite pearls), Sabine, Sarah and Tarryn. I am also deeply grateful to those who entrusted me with their stories.

To my family and friends for your constant support and encouragement. Mum, thanks for having me and showing me how to nurture myself. To all the women before me for lighting the way, and to Queen Constance for your seal of approval. Finally, to my husband for your endless love, lucidity, positivity and musculature. Thanks for taking care of me in every phase.

INDEX